D1105275

Reboot Your Body

21-Day
Detox Program

Dr. Said Sokhandan

Published by Dr. Said Sokhandan, Mukilteo, Washington

Printed in the United States

Library of Congress Cataloging-in-Publications Data
Sokhandan, Said
  Reboot Your Body : 21 Day Detox Program / by Dr. Said Sokhandan. Edited by Theresa Poalucci
  1. Naturopathic Detox Program

Library of Congress Control Number: 2010935153

To the one person whom I owe everything, my wife, Maryam Sokhandan. Her unwavering faith and confidence is what has shaped me to be the person I am today.

Acknowledgments

As with any major project, it doesn't happen without the help of other people. My book is no different. I am grateful for the help of the following people.

I'll begin by thanking Carolyn Johnson, Mariah Oehling and Helen Kendal for their participation as test readers. I sincerely appreciate their feedback and contributions to this effort.

Andrew Ballard helped in launching this project with market research, positioning and promotion recommendations. I also want to wholeheartedly thank my editor, Theresa Poalucci; I could not have completed this book without her time, talent and direction.

And of course I thank my wife Maryam for putting up with all of the late nights I spent researching and writing this book. My thanks also go out to my beloved mother who showed me the true love and patience.

Finally, I would like to take the opportunity to thank all my teachers and mentors.

Table of Contents

Forward

On perusing this book, it will come as no surprise to the reader that Said Sokhandan was an architect before he became a physician The text is developed in such a way that the content is a framework built upon a foundation. That framework, in turn, supports a structure that the reader will want to inhabit.

The foundation is Sokhandan's view of health—that it is not a commodity to be acquired from a practitioner but a responsibility to be nurtured by every human being. Such persons are not considered "patients" to be treated so much as "agents" of their own health in a world where the physician is a teacher who imparts education. This education empowers the person to eat, exercise and live responsibly and in such a way as to engender health rather than invite disease.

The framework is the set of scientific and practical assumptions upon which a healthy life may be structured.

Based on sound science and reflecting keen insight into the influence of environmental issues and dietary practices, Sokhandan charts a course to health, making understandable the complex interactions among human biology, natural products and pharmaceutical agents.

Dr. Sokhandan's work is accessible in style, practical in content and encouraging in its tone. He writes with a sincere and tender regard for the welfare of the reader, making himself vulnerable from time to time by using illustrations from his own life experience. In this way, his counsel seems welcome and easy to embrace. The anecdotes from his clinical practice provide further reason for our paying attention to his advice. I commend this work to you.

Daniel K. Church, PhD
President
Bastyr University

About Dr. Said Sokhandan

Doctor S (Said Sokhandan, N.D.) is a Naturopathic physician as a Primary Care Provider, licensed in the State of Washington.

Additional specializations: Dr. S has extensive post-graduate training in variety of holistic therapeutic, homo-toxicology (detoxification), anti-aging, and diagnostic techniques. Herbal Medicine - Acupuncture and Integrated Nutritional Counseling.

Dr. Said Sokhandan first became interested in medicine through his grandmother, who herself was a naturopath. "When I was young," says Dr. Sokhandan, "I was fascinated that villagers came from so far away to see her." His grandmother's example eventually led him to complete a Doctoral degree in Naturopathic Medicine at Bastyr University. He also has a Master of Science in acupuncture and oriental medicine, and was trained at the Shanghai University Research Institute. He is licensed as a Primary Care Provider by the State of Washington.

How Naturopathy Is Different

Traditional western medicine tends to begin by looking at isolated body parts—heart, stomach, nerves, etc., and to focus on medications as the treatment of choice. A naturopathic physician focuses on the person as a whole, not just the parts. Besides examining the physical body, Dr. Sokhandan also takes into account a person's mental, emotional, and spiritual condition. While he is licensed to prescribe medication when appropriate, it may often be a treatment of last resort. Naturopathy is enjoying revived popularity as people begin to understand its possibilities, and insurance companies begin to open up to naturopathic treatments.

"In Western medicine, everything is being prescribed these days, from Viagra to Prozac," Dr. Sokhandan says. "But society is becoming more educated, and we're trying to assist by being teachers. We want to help you learn what is good for your own body and your personal circumstances. Then you'll be better able to take care of yourself."

It's Your Life

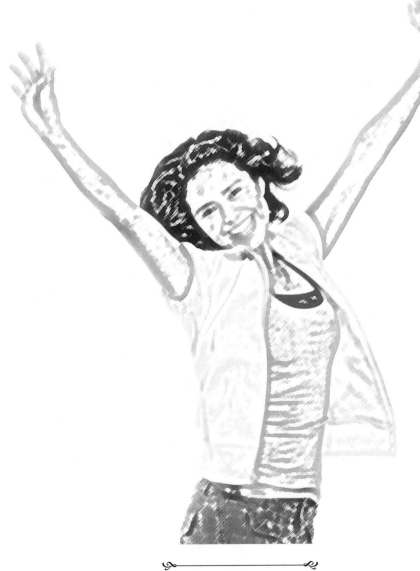

It's Your Life

This is a book about you. It is about your health and well-being. It is about improving your situation, even while living in a mostly man-made and complicated world. Reading this book could possibly change your life. It could possibly lengthen your life. It could save your life.

How much do you know about your body? What is missing in your life?

If you get up in the morning with no energy, craving coffee, worried about everyone except you, feeling stressed or emotional, or worried about relationships — shouldn't you take care of yourself first? How can you really solve problems or take care of others when you are in this state of mind?

Think about what is affecting your body and well-being. This book is a guide to help you understand how you can take the steps necessary to acquire optimum health.

You may have heard claims from others about how to be healthy; stop here! You are responsible for your own health. This is a guide that will give you the tools to take the steps necessary to help you build a better you. You will learn about your body, about what you digest and what it does to you, about how to get rid of the toxins that are certainly already there, about allergies that you may not even know you have (both food and environmental), and about how to avoid feeling poorly in the future. You will need to be ready to pretox, detox, and protox. You will learn what is toxic, how to read food labels, what vitamins and minerals do, the importance of cooking properly, about toxins in the home and workplace, and how to maintain balance.

Why Trust Me?

Since I will be addressing the most important subject, you, let me start by telling you a little about me, in the interest of gaining your trust and perhaps your friendship.

I did not become a naturopathic physician (ND) until I had first become successful in different careers, as an entrepreneur, an architect, and a chef. For me and my family, it was a leap of faith to disrupt our comfortable lives so that I could pursue my dream of studying medicine — a goal I felt compelled to achieve.

While attending school, I found myself constantly questioning standard medical practices. So once I was licensed, I continued to study, eventually mastering Chinese medical practices and homeopathic medicine to enhance the care I could offer patients. I now practice a mixture of all that I have mastered and believe about how to attain and retain optimum health.

I have an office in a suburb just north of Seattle. My patients, for the most part, need to be treated for problems that could have been avoided. Whether their symptoms stem from what they eat, what they are exposed to in their environment, over-work and no play, or a genetic make-up that predisposes them to a specific problem, they always come looking for a quick fix.

Modern medicine is a miracle, but often general practitioners are overwhelmed with the demands of seeing a high number of patients each hour. These doctors must also deal with the requirements of a massive disassociated health insurance web that can often have them spending more time on paperwork than with their patients. The bottom line is that for many doctors, the easiest answer is to prescribe a pill and send their patients on their way.

My patients will tell you that walking away with a prescription for whatever the most fashionable new wonder drug is from my office is rare. I don't even carry a prescription pad in my pocket, nor do I have one placed on every desk in every examination room. I'm not saying that there isn't a time or place. For example, I am currently treating a young woman who was diagnosed as bipolar. When she came to see me she was taking nine separate prescriptions, yet could not function normally. She now takes the one prescription that she needs. Her life is back on track.

Many drugs, even over-the-counter medicines, can cause harmful side effects when they interact with each other or are used improperly. Others can be dangerous when combined with alcohol, caffeine, and even certain foods. In fact, few people realize that some drugs even cancel each other out when taken together or with certain vitamins, minerals, or foods.

The adage, "no pain, no gain," certainly will be true if you decide to turn your health around in the ways that I am going to suggest — ways that are natural and do not include prescription drugs. High blood

If you think that a pill is the answer, you might consider that one of every 31 hospitalizations in this country results from an adverse drug reaction (ADR). More than 2.2 million ADRs result in more than 100,000 deaths per year among hospitalized patients. Some studies venture that ADRs are the fourth leading cause of death — ahead of pulmonary disease, diabetes, AIDS, pneumonia, accidents, and automobile deaths.

You might also consider that over half of all medications are used incorrectly. In fact, while Americans spend about $77 billion a year on prescriptions, over $76 billion is spent to treat problems that result from improper use of drugs, adverse reactions, and drug interactions. If you are like most people, you've taken prescription drugs, and you've likely taken more than one drug at the same time. You probably also take drugs now and then that you buy without a prescription — like pain relievers, cough, cold, and allergy medicines.

pressure, diabetes, depression, digestive problems, headaches, and more are symptoms of a much larger problem — how you are living your life, and more accurately, what you are ingesting every day.

I am going to share with you a regimen which has proven itself over and over again in my practice with the myriad of patients I have treated. Yes, it requires some sacrifice, but the rewards far outweigh the inconvenience.

Is a longer, healthier life worth giving up certain foods and changing a few things in your environment? If you didn't answer the question with a resounding yes, then let me give you a few reasons why you should be ready to enact change.

Your body is a toxic waste land

If you do not clean it often, the body will die.

We are in contact with toxic chemicals every day which seep into our bodies through a variety of products, from food additives, to the water we drink, to the pesticides we ingest, and even from the cosmetics we use. We are bombarded with man-made chemicals everywhere. Just consider the fact that, according to a government study, we spend an average of 15 hours a day at home surrounded by materials filled with synthetic chemical compounds. With more than 80,000 chemicals used in the United States and 2,000 new compounds being introduced every year, the average American is exposed to a cocktail of unnatural substances every day.

This unnatural mix of chemicals can be detected by blood and urine tests in your doctor's office, but why do the test if you don't have the ability to fix the problem? Tests show that the average person living in the modern world will have up to 85% synthetic chemicals in their system. These toxins can cause any number of physical problems, such as degenerative and more rapid aging, and ailments ranging from allergies to cancer. The body's natural ability to cleanse itself internally can become overloaded with these toxic residues. When this occurs, the body's cells can't work at peak efficiency, which sets off a domino effect for potential health problems.

Everyone is exposed to two types of toxins. Exotoxins are toxins that originate outside the body. They might include mercury from fillings, pollutants in the air, or the use of cleansers or compounds you are exposed to at work.

Interestingly, children have been found to have twice the levels of toxins in their blood than adults, simply from playing with soft plastic toys.

The other type are endotoxins, which originate from the daily work of the body's cells. Endotoxins are normally released by the body through waste and sweat, but if there is over-saturation, this type of toxin can cause blockage of the bile duct, inflammation, liver damage, and the production of free radicals.

Some chemicals can accumulate in the body faster than others, such as dioxins, which are often found in fast foods or foods cooked in the microwave in a plastic container. Dioxins are highly poisonous to our cells and cause cancer, especially breast cancer (according to a study conducted by Johns Hopkins University). High exposure to dioxins have been linked to mood alterations, reduced cognitive performance, diabetes, lessening of the immune system, endometriosis, decreased fertility, decreased testosterone levels, and elevated thyroxin levels.

Other toxins that exist in the environment such as pesticides, fungi, bacteria, viruses, and allergens can have a negative effect on both the immune system and endocrine system. Hydrocarbons, formaldehyde, the compounds in cleaning products, ozone, carbon dioxide, and vehicle emissions accumulate in the body daily and all will have an effect on our overall health. Heavy metal toxicity like arsenic, cadmium, and mercury buildup will stay in the body as these are difficult for the body to excrete. Accumulated heavy metal toxicity can cause injury to the cell structure of the vascular system. This process will cause depletion and inactivation of minerals such as selenium, zinc, and glutathione, all essential to good health.

The body is not able to metabolize many of the toxins we ingest or are exposed to. The elimination of certain chemicals is so slow that it can take many years before they vacate a body. In the meantime these toxins remain for years in our blood, fat tissue (adipose), semen, muscle, bone, brain tissue, and other organs. Chlorinated water and pesticides such as DDT can remain in the body for 50 years — while arsenic, for example (which we are exposed to through detergent, car exhaust, and pesticides), is mostly excreted within 72 hours of exposure. Whether chemicals quickly pass through or are stored in the body, they still remain a burden to our systems.

How many of the approximately 80,000 chemicals that are used in the United States can one body withstand?

You can't stop living in the world, but you can change what you put in your mouth!

Grow up in the U.S. and you grow up eating fast food, sweets, white bread, and a host of other edibles that taste good and even make you feel good for a short period of time. No one ever thinks of the possible health effects that eating these kinds of foods will have later in life.

Since I have now had years of experience working with my patients and have become proficient on the subject of the human body, not only on a physical level but also taking into account the emotional aspects of a person, I have come to believe that our food must be nutritious for optimum health and well-being. Food today isn't what it was for our grandparents, or to a certain degree for our parents. In the past 40 years, large corporations have become the owners of the food industry and they have changed our eating habits dramatically.

Most of the foods we consume today contain chemicals and coloring agents, emulsifiers, and thickeners simply to improve their appearance. Artificial preservatives are added to increase the shelf life of what we eat. For better flavor, chemical enhancers are now used in the manufacturing of food, as well as processing agents to keep food products consistent during production. Non-organic vitamins and minerals are added to increase nutritional values. Since the FDA does not closely control foods that have no nutritional value, it is our personal responsibility to take charge of what we eat by looking at the nutritional values listed on the label and reading between the lines. Nutritional values are often not really valuable. In a later chapter you will learn how to tell the difference.

I see a lot of patients with symptoms such as high blood pressure, high cholesterol, gout, and central obesity (where fat deposits are mainly around the waist, also known as metabolic syndrome x). Over time these conditions will damage cells so that they no longer can properly utilize insulin, converting glucose to energy. In a healthy person the average insulin receptor site per cell is up to 20,000, while the individual with metabolic syndrome x tests at as few as 5,000. Since glucose in the bloodstream becomes the job of the liver, to clear from the blood, it turns the glucose to fat. The end results could be diabetes or cancer.

Genetic factors also play a role in insulin resistance. Some people, for instance, can have a pancreas that overproduces insulin. However for the majority of us, it is all about what we are ingesting at the dinner table. Adding what we eat to the constant attack by toxins in our environment, it is not hard to understand why we have so many health problems.

The Benefits
of Detox

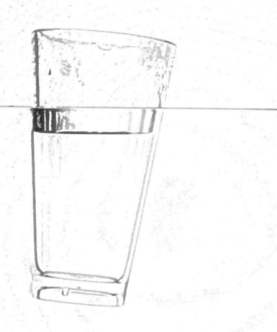

The benefits of detox?
The body does this daily.

If you were perfectly healthy, your body would detox itself every day. If the body becomes overwhelmed and cannot detox itself naturally, then the process of cell reproduction is compromised and that spells big trouble. Over-saturation means the body cannot detox fast enough, and it starts to make choices about what it needs to take care of first. Let's say you are fighting a cold. Your body will fight the cold and leave toxins alone in other parts of the body. Let's say you ate too much at a turkey dinner and you have too much to digest. Some of what you ate will stay with you longer than it should.

I tell my patients that they need to detox their bodies two times a year, much like they see their dentist for a cleaning. Even though you brush and floss every day, you still make that extra effort. Your body needs the same type of maintenance.

Why?

▸▸ More than one-third of the individuals born in the U.S. in the year 2000 are expected to develop diabetes.
▸▸ In 2008, 64.5% of Americans were overweight and 30.5% were obese.
▸▸ Prevalence of depression and age-adjusted prevalence of osteoporosis are increasing.
▸▸ Congestive heart failure increased by 118% from 1979 to 1992.
▸▸ Migraine prevalence increased from 1980 to 1989.
▸▸ Asthma increased 75% from 1980 to 1999.

And if you don't think these statistics are affecting your pocketbook, think again. There has been a double-digit increase in

Toxic effects of white flour

Some foods like white flour are nutritionally devastating for the human body and should be limited in consumption. White flour can actually deplete the body of needed vitamins and minerals. Just take a look at the chart below:

White flour depletes these vitamins:

Thiamine (B1).................. 77 %
Riboflavin (B2)................. 80 %
Niacin (B3) .... 82 %
Pantothenate (B5)............. 50 %
Vitamin (B6)...................... 72 %
Vitamin E .... 86 %
Betaine .... 23 %
Choline .... 30 %

White flour depletes these minerals:

Magnesium .... 85 %
Calcium............................. 60 %
Potassium .... 77 %
Chromium .... 40 %
Manganese .... 86 %
Selenium........................... 16 %
Iron................................... 76 %
Copper .... 68 %
Zinc .... 78 %

The chart is just one example of a common food you probably consume every day. Consider these facts before you sit down to your next meal.

insurance premiums each year for the past five consecutive years, starting with 2003. The number of Americans without medical insurance has reached 43.6 million. More than one million bankruptcies in 2007 were attributed to medical issues. Increasing growth of the Medicare-eligible population will raise overall costs of the Medicare program from $271 billion in 2003 to $3.9 trillion in 2013.

A little knowledge can go a long way

Before I lay out the detox program for you, you are going to have to learn about the various components that make up what you eat. You have to be schooled enough to read the label at the grocery store and determine whether or not the food is good or bad for you. I always tell my patients the fewer ingredients listed the better.

Take, for example, bread the way grandma used to make it, flour water, salt, and yeast. Today a bread label reads more like a chemistry book.

You can see from the above sample that what various vitamins and minerals can do is important, as is how they can be depleted by eating certain foods. As part of the detox program, I will be suggesting you supplement your food intake with nutrients that can help you through the process in a most amazing way. My patients tell me that they don't feel like they are starving, nor are they craving sugar or other items they have eliminated from their diet during the detox process.

Sound too good to be true? Let me give you a couple of true case examples.

I recently treated a 48-year-old male executive whose chief complaints included heartburn, high cholesterol, osteoporosis (due to medication for heartburn), and a weight issue. He took several prescribed medications.

His blood work showed his cholesterol level was 354, triglyceride was 287 and LDL was 244. These levels respectively should have been under 200, under 100, and under 100.

This man's fasting blood sugar came in at 115. For his age it should have been 80 to 85. The blood work report showed that his body leaned toward being acidic, a situation which made him even more prone to toxicity and disease.

After three weeks of detoxifying, nudging him toward some simple lifestyle changes, and taking away his medication, his

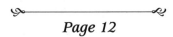

cholesterol dropped to 198, triglyceride to 129, and LDL went to 124. His blood sugar at fasting was 110 and his hemoglobin told me he was no longer pre-diabetic as well. Before detox his weight was 176 pounds, and his body fat was 30.4%. After detox his body weight had dropped to 152 pounds, and his body fat was 27%. This patient has told me that he now feels in control of his health for the first time in his life, and he is pleased to be off his prescribed medications. Further, he no longer worries about heartburn.

At 51 years old, a female teacher who had recently moved to Washington from Arizona came to see me with a laundry list of tough problems. She had been diagnosed as suffering from bipolar mania, asthma, hypothyroidism, irritable bowel syndrome (IBS), and she was overweight. She also was complaining of pain in her fingers, hands, knees, and legs. In fact, the pain in her legs would wake her up at night. I also observed she had a rash on her forehead, face, and neck. To add to her traumas, she suffered from night sweats and hot flashes.

She described her mood swings as being the most difficult when she first went to bed. She said she felt every wrinkle in the sheets and could not get comfortable. This patient felt like a prisoner in her own body.

She had given up the profession she loved, teaching, because of her health issues. None of her primary care physicians could make a sound diagnosis and she was on a myriad of medications, which seemed to increase every time she visited the doctor's office. By the time she came to see me, she was on nine different medications. I asked how she had been treated by her primary caregivers and what type of blood work they had done on her, but her communication skills were very poor at the time and I did not learn much.

After a long history intake, we did a complete blood work-up including examining hormone levels. Her blood work showed she was suffering from low levels of estrogen, progesterone, and testosterone. Her body toxicity was high. After eight weeks of a complete lifestyle change and a detox program in which I added some much needed nutrients and hormones back into her system naturally, she became communicative once again, feels healthy, and is back to her first love, teaching.

A final example I would like to share with you concerns a 67-year-old man who was against taking any kind of medication, yet he was about to become a diabetic and had high blood pressure. His regular physician sent him to me for natural remedies for his various health issues.

Here is a sample of a portion of his blood work when he first came to see me:

Glucose .... value 101 .... range 65-99 (mg/dL)
Cholesterol .... value 265 .... range 150-240 (mg/dL)
HDL Cholesterol ..... value 55 ...... range 40-70 (mg/dL)
LDL Cholesterol ..... value 180 .... range 3-130 (mg/dL)

Here is a sample of a portion of his blood work after just four weeks of detox:

Glucose .... value 86 ...... range 65-99 (mg/dL)
Cholesterol .... value 184 .... range 150-240 (mg/dL)
HDL Cholesterol ..... value 38 ...... range 40-70 (mg/dL)
LDL Cholesterol ..... value 132 .... range 3-130 (mg/dL)

From the blood work, you can see that this man, in just four weeks, avoided diabetes, a possible heart attack, or stroke, or both.

These three examples may sound dramatic, but they are an everyday occurrence in my office. Both of these patients, and many others, had to first learn about what would bring them to optimum health. They needed to detoxify. They had to make a commitment to arm themselves with the knowledge required to make good choices. They had to make some changes, but I would expect that both of them would tell you it was well worth it.

So how does what you eat affect you? Let's look at the basics.

Function of Proteins, Amino Acids, and Carbohydrates

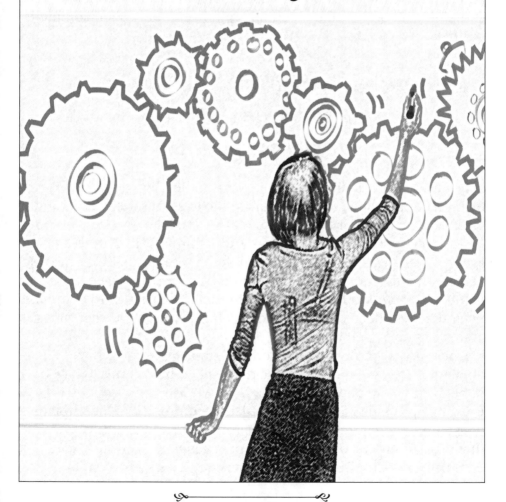

Function of proteins in the body

Protein is one of the necessary components for human body growth and repair. Protein is also essential in making and maintaining enzymes, antibodies, and blood. The human body needs 22 amino acids. Of the 22 necessary, nine cannot be made by the body and are called essential amino acids. The body manufactures the other 13 non-essential amino acids. Foods containing all of the nine essential amino acids are called complete proteins.

Protein is second only to water as the most essential element that makes up the body.

Protein is the building block for our muscles, ligaments, tendons, teeth, nails, and skin. It is also part of the enzymes, hormones, and antibodies needed for the body to maintain health.

Complete proteins usually come from animal-based foods such as meat, fish, eggs, and dairy. Incomplete proteins are those missing some of the essential amino acids and therefore must be eaten in combination with other foods, within a 24 hour period, to complete what the body needs. Incomplete proteins are found in vegetables, grains, legumes, and nuts.

Since meats, poultry, dairy products, and eggs tend to have all nine of the essential amino acids we need from foods, what happens if you are a vegetarian or a vegan? You must depend on vegetable proteins. Just because vegetable proteins are incomplete doesn't mean that they are less healthy or nutritious. It turns out that if you combine different types of vegetables, you can create complete proteins. Complete proteins can also be achieved by combining certain foods with amino acid supplements. We know this works as many vegetarian-based cultures have been combining vegetable proteins for thousands of years.

There is one exception to the rule about protein in vegetables and it can be found in soybeans. Soybeans are one of the few vegetable sources that contain complete protein in nature. Many Asian cultures have made soybeans an essential part of their diet. Tofu is concentrated soy protein that is made from soybeans and is a meat alternative which contains all nine.

How much protein do we need? Most healthy eating guides recommend between 10-15% of daily calories come from protein; however, protein needs can change dramatically during different life stages. During some stages of life such as puberty, pregnancy, while breast-feeding, during heavy exercise, or illness, a body may need significantly more protein every day.

Most Americans consume more than enough protein, and since it is abundant in many foods, you shouldn't have to worry about not getting enough. But, just as in the case of fat, you should avoid eating too much protein. You should also pay attention to the quality or type of protein you consume.

In nature, protein and fat are closely tied together. In most foods, complete proteins (like in animal products or tofu products) are almost always high in fat. Therefore when eating meats or poultry, recognized as a "high-protein foods," realize that you are most likely eating a lot of fat as well. In contrast, plant proteins are much lower in fat and also rich in fiber and nutrients. When combined together, grains, legumes, nuts, and seeds become the real "high-protein foods" with the added benefit of being low in fat.

Examples of good high protein foods:
Eggs • Milk • Soy • Wheat
Meats (including beef, chicken, and fish)

Amino acids

Most people lack the proper amount of amino acids in their systems and they don't even know it. Amino acids are the building blocks of our cells — the main constituents that make up protein. While a carbohydrate can provide a cell with energy, it is the amino acids that allow a cell to grow and maintain structure.

Amino acids can be attributed to energy, the body's ability to recover, muscle strength, fat loss, and brain function. When the digestive system is weak or does not have the proper amino acids because of toxins from the wrong kind of diet, exposure to harmful chemicals in the environment, stress, or a lack of enzymes, then you have a situation that is ripe for disease to begin.

Dietary amino acids are

You can't lose weight by exercise alone

If someone tells you that all you need to do to lose weight is go to the gym, tell them to prove it. Hand them your gym card, pat them on the back and give them an encouraging smile, then tell them to knock themselves out. One rule — they can't change their eating habits.

Exercise will help prevent obesity, but it won't make you lose weight. Being fit and being thin are not synonymous. Take a weight lifter for instance. He may be able to bench press a couple hundred pounds, but I bet he can't run a marathon. The marathon runner probably can't bench press a lot of weight. And both of them are still in danger of diabetes or heart disease if they aren't watchful of what they ingest.

Walk, bike, or swim and you help your cardiovascular system and respiratory system. Lift weights or do resistance training and you will build muscles. Build up a good sweat and you get rid of toxins. But most people fool themselves into thinking that it is OK to eat that donut because, after all they exercised.

To be physically fit means that you are able to increase agility and gain stamina through practice. It makes everyday movement easier and you can increase your coordination. Staying active is by all means mandatory for overall good health, but it will never replace the benefits of ridding your body of toxins and then being vigilante about eating only safe and natural foods.

Some doctors have argued that over doing exercise may actually be harmful and I don't mean the obvious, such as to many years of running can wreck your knees. I am talking about the fact that research has shown that when you exercise heavily (in spurts), your body sends hunger signals and you simply overeat after these episodes. Not only do you eat more, but usually much more than the calories you actually burned. It takes a lot of strenuous activity to burn the calories of say a sugar donut.

A popular national donut chain reports 190 calories in their sugar donut, 80 of these calories are from fat. You would need to walk for one-

normally consumed in the form of proteins which are broken down into individual amino acids by the digestive system and then are re-synthesized into endogenous proteins (works in the system for cell energy). All amino acids are white, crystalline, and soluble in water. They are called amino acids because they all contain an amino group (NH2) and a carboxyl group (COOH), which is acidic.

Individual amino acids (there are 23) are usually classified according to their importance in providing an essential part of the diet and are also classified according to their chemical structure.

Why do you need to know about the different kinds of amino acids? Well, you wouldn't take an aspirin to stop bleeding and you wouldn't eat Rolaids for a headache, would you? Then it is important to know what the amino acids in your food may or may not be doing for you. Here are the groups:

▸▸ Acidic amino acids are a group of amino acids with a side chain also containing an acidic group. They facilitate the growth of blood vessels, form heart muscle, stimulate proliferation, differentiate spleen tissue, increase thymus gland weight, and enhance the function of the thymus gland (for your immune system). Acidic amino acids also improve the function of thyroid glands, eliminate fatigue, protect the liver from certain toxins, strengthen bones and teeth, and are a source of energy in the brain.

▸▸ Basic amino acids have a side chain containing a basic group. This group of amino acids inhibits the primary mechanism of the aging process (cross-linking, which you will learn about later in this book). Basic

hour, swim for thrity-minutes, or you could cut that in half again by rowing for fifteen minutes.

Another problem with the gym work out is the risk to your self-control. Exercise and you get hungry, The hungrier you are the harder it is not to eat, especially sugar, which most of us crave after a strenuous workout.

Then there is the problem of your energy level. If you are truly curbing your calories to lose weight, then you don't want to use up all your energy in one hour at the gym. Rather a slow and steady day of continuing activity might serve you and your diet more effectively.

Here is a list of what it takes to work off what you eat. Numbers are based on a weight of 180 pounds and 30 minute of activity:

• Aerobics - 162 calories

• Baseball - 140 calories

• Walking the dog - 118 calories

• Housecleaning - 172 calories

• Mowing lawn - 130 calories

• Stair climbing - 244 calories

• Tennis (doubles) - 137 calories

amino acids decrease hardening of the arteries, improve blood circulation, prevent abnormal blood clotting, lower blood pressure, reduce intestinal permeability, alleviate certain types of colitis, prevent bacterial and viral diseases, block some forms of cancer, relieve inflammation, and reduce insulin resistance.

▶▶ Branched chain amino acids (BCAAs) are a group of amino acids with a branched side chain. The term branched chain arises from the fact that BCAAs have aliphatic side chains that are non-linear. These are leucine, isoleucine, and valine. These are considered essential amino acids because we as humans cannot survive unless these amino acids are present in the diet. For example, isoleucine is required for the creation of hemoglobin, alleviates hypoglycemia, facilitates muscle growth, and is essential for optimal skin function.

▶▶ Essential amino acids are necessary for the maintenance of human health and must be supplied via the diet, as the body cannot manufacture them from other amino acids. Essential amino acids are precursors for the endogenous synthesis of non-essential amino acids within the liver. They consist of (a) isoleucine, (b) leucine, (c) lysine, (d) methionine, (e) phenylalanine, (f) threonine, (g) tryptophan, (h) valine, and (i) histidine.

▶▶ Glucogenic amino acids form metabolic intermediates, which form glucose after they have lost their amino group (usually by transmigration). Glucogenic amino acids facilitate the body's production of energy (after they have been metabolized to glucose within the liver). This conversion is catalyzed by glucagon (a hormone). This group of amino acids consists of (a) alanine, (b) arginine, (c) aspartic acid, (d) cysteine, (e) glutamic acid, (f) glycine, (g) histidine, (h) methionine, (i) phenylalanine, (j) proline, (k) serine, (l) threonine, (m) tyrosine, and (n) valine. For example, alanine is essential for the correct function of the adrenal gland, is a component of the cell wall of good intestinal bacteria, enhances brain function, and alleviates epilepsy in some patients.

▸▸ Ketogenic amino acids form ketones after losing their amino group. They are (a) leucine, (b) phenylalanine, and (c) tyrosine. For example, leucine stabilizes elevated blood sugar, which is utilized for the production of energy and released from muscle for exercise, and facilitates recovery of skeletal muscle after exercise.

▸▸ Large neutral amino acids are comparatively large but neutral molecules that share a common transport method through the blood-brain barrier and therefore compete with each other for entry into the brain. They are (a) isoleucine, (b) leucine, (c) phenylalanine, (d) tryptophan, (e) tyrosine, and (f) valine. For example, tryptophan stimulates the production of antibodies, suppresses inflammation for patients with fibromialga, reduces aggressiveness by stimulating the production of serentonin, helps reduce anxiety, helps with bulimia and anorexia, stops cravings of carbohydrates, and alleviates insomnia, headaches, and migraines.

▸▸ Non-essential amino acids are not deemed to be important constituents of the human diet as they can be synthesized from essential amino acids. Non-essential amino acids can be synthesized within the liver from essential amino acids. This group consists of (a) alanine, (b) arginine, (c) asparagine, (d) aspartic acid, (e) citrulline, (f) cysteine, (g) cystine, (h) glutamic acid, (i) glycine, (j) histidine, (k) serine, and (l) tyrosine.

▸▸ Sulfuric amino acids are amino acids that include sulfur in their chemical structure. These consist of (a) cysteine, (b) cystine, (c) methionine, and (d) taurine. For example, cystine comprises 8% of human hair, prevents damage of hair follicles, helps prevent some forms of cancer, is a potent antioxidant, deactivates certain free radicals, enhances function of the thyroid gland, decreases inflammation for rheumatoid arthritis, and prevents fatty liver from alcohol.

▸▸ Urea cycle amino acids facilitate the excretion of ammonia (formed from the breakdown of the endogenous nitrogen derived from "spent" amino acids) from the body via urea. They are (a) arginine, (b) citrulline, and (c) ornithine. Ornithine, for example, stimulates the immune system, enhances regeneration of the liver, and is useful for the treatment of Alzheimer's disease.

Function of carbohydrates in the body

The main function of carbohydrates is to provide a substrate for the production of energy in the body, and heat. After conversion to glucose, it is stored until needed. Carbohydrates facilitate tryptophan's entry into the brain (remember your list of amino acids). Remember after grandma's turkey dinner, how you felt like taking a nap? That was caused by tryptophan.

There are two types of carbohydrates: simple and complex. Simple carbohydrates consist of a group of simple sugars which accelerate the aging process and can cause depression, anxiety, hypertension, or irritable bowel syndrome. A complex carbohydrate is a polysaccharide which can increase energy, essential in the production of saturated fatty acids, and it is important for digestion.

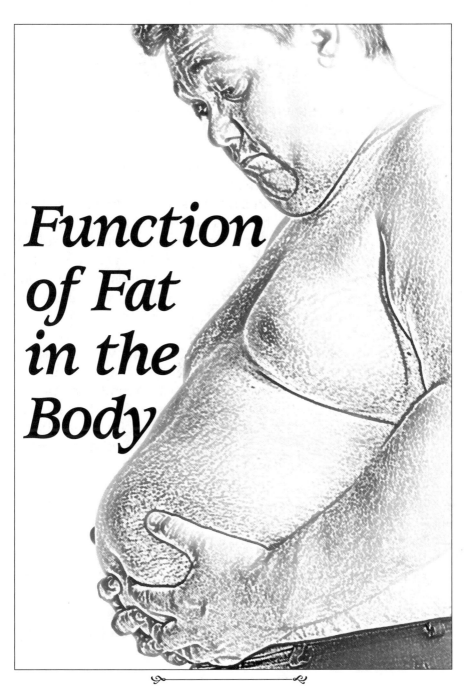

Function of Fat in the Body

Function of fat in the body

Fat is a substrate for energy production. Due to a lack of proper knowledge, our society has become "fat-phobic," and many popular diet programs completely discourage the consumption of fat in their programs. However, any reasonable doctor will tell you that some fat does have a place in a healthy body.

Before getting into the technical details of fat, here is a brief list of some of the beneficial roles fat plays in our diet. Fat provides energy to our cells and is needed to circulate, store, and absorb fat-soluble vitamins such as A, D, E, and K. Fat supplies the raw materials to make some of the hormones and other compounds needed in your body, and fat promotes healthy skin and hair. Fat provides a layer of insulation and protection around your vital organs like your kidneys and heart as well.

Of course, like any food product, too much of anything can lead to health problems, and fat is no exception. North Americans tend to consume too many fatty foods and processed foods, and that can lead to serious health problems like heart disease, strokes, diabetes, and cancer. When a scientist or doctor refers to a fat, they usually use the word triglyceride. This is the general term used to describe the main form of fat in food and in the body.

A triglyceride is made up of a 3-carbon "backbone," called glycerol, that has three (i.e. tri-) fatty acid chains attached to it. These fatty acids are long chains of carbon atoms with hydrogen attached, and their structure is what determines the beneficial or harmful properties of the fat.

Apart from eating too much fat, most people eat the wrong kind of fat, because all fats are NOT created equal. Fat comes in a variety of types, with some being more harmful than others. In addition to watching your total fat intake, you have to pay attention to the type of fat you eat.

Monounsaturated fats

When most of the fatty acid chains in the triglyceride molecule have only one double bond, the fat is called monounsaturated (i.e. one spot is not saturated). Olive oils, canola oils, peanut oils, sesame seed oils, avocados, and most nuts are high in monounsaturated fat. The latest research shows that these types of fat are the most beneficial for you when eaten in moderation. Eating too much will not provide more benefits and will load you up with fat calories.

Polyunsaturated fats

Where monounsaturated has one double bond in the fatty acid chains, polyunsaturated fat has two or more double bonds (i.e. two or more spots are not saturated). Most vegetable oils like corn oils, safflower oils, sunflower oils, and soybean oils are polyunsaturated. These oils are beneficial if eaten in moderation, but not when they are used for frying. Unfortunately, most fast foods are deep fried in polyunsaturated oils, making them especially bad if consumed in excess.

Essential fatty acids

There are two types of polyunsaturated fat, called essential fatty acids, that we absolutely need to get from our food. The essential fatty acids we know come in two types and are called omega-6 and omega-3. Most people get enough omega-6 from vegetable oils, but don't get enough omega-3 fatty acids. These beneficial types of fat are not used in the body as calories; instead, they are used as building blocks in the body to make hormones, neurotransmitters, and other cellular components. The best sources of essential fatty acids include unprocessed whole nuts and seeds, especially flax seeds. They're also found in larger quantities in cold water fish like salmon, tuna, mackerel, anchovies, and sardines but are destroyed when the foods are fried in oil. The lesson? Go for fish, but not fried fish & chips!

How much fat should we eat?

Most health care professionals recommend that less than 30% of the day's total calories should come from fat, and less than 10% of the day's total calories should come from saturated fat. This works out to be about 65 grams of fat per day for a 2000 calorie diet. But this figure is only an estimate — some people do better with significantly higher or lower amounts of healthy fats in their daily diet. How much you need should be determined by your health care professional.

Saturated fatty acids

Saturated fatty acids are the simplest types of fatty acids. They carry a carboxyl (acid) group at one end and the rest of the molecule is fatty material. The fatty material is an arrangement of carbon atoms chained together, and each of the remaining positions on the carbon atoms are filled (saturated) by hydrogen atoms. Saturated fatty acid carbon chains are from two to 28 carbon atoms long. Saturated fatty acids contain no double bonds, are slow to react with other chemicals, and carry no electrical charges.

Saturated fatty acids are differentiated from unsaturated fatty acids by the absence of double bonds in their chemical structure. Saturated fatty acids are a component of cell membranes and are commonly found in animal products, like flesh foods and dairy. They are the most harmful type of fat when eaten in excess but are still an important part of the diet. North Americans consume too much saturated fat, in the form of meats, processed foods, and desserts like ice-cream and chocolate.

Types of saturated fatty acids

➤ Short chain saturated fatty acids that contain four to six carbon atoms are utilized primarily in the production of energy. The two types of short chain fatty acids are (a) butyric acid and (b) caproic acid.

➤ Medium chain saturated fatty acids contain eight to 12 carbon atoms and are mainly used within the body to produce energy and help to prevent and treat obesity. The types of medium chain are (a) caprylic acid, (b) capric acid, and (c) lauric acid.

➤ Long chain saturated fatty acids contain 14 to 24 carbon atoms, are essentially toxic, and should be avoided. Types of long chain are (a) arachidic acid, (b) behenic acid, (c) lignoceric acid, (d) myristic acid, (e) palmitic acid, (f) pentadecanoic acid, and (g) stearic acid.

Excessive consumption of long chain saturated fatty acids increases the risk of atherosclerosis, diabetes, stroke, heart attack, blood clotting, and obesity.

Trans fatty acids (or partially hydrogenated vegetable oil)

This type of fat is not found in nature but is created during a process called hydrogenation. Partial-hydrogenation is an industrial process that utilizes hydrogen gas at high temperatures to modify the unsaturated fatty acids found in dietary plant oils into mutated substances that are commercially easier to package and market.

The food industry uses this process to make the fat more stable in their food products or to change its properties. Partial-hydrogenation converts the structure of the unsaturated fatty acids in dietary oils to highly toxic trans fatty acids. Margarine is made by hydrogenating vegetable oils into a spreadable solid form that is high in trans fatty acids. Since trans fats do not occur in nature, our bodies are not designed to handle them very well and use them like saturated fats in our bodies. This is not good news, since saturated fats are the most harmful type of fat, and North Americans tend to consume too much anyway.

Trans fatty acids are present in foods containing traditional stick margarine, bakery and frying fats, vegetable shortenings, and margarine that have been subjected to hydrogenation. They have now become a universal food culture and are readily reflected in bakery products and other packaged snacks such as microwave popcorn, fried foods, and breakfast margarine and, to a smaller extent, in dairy and meat products. In today's world, it is almost impossible to eliminate trans fats completely, so the best thing to do is reduce the amount of processed foods you eat, and limit products that have the words "hydrogenated" or "partially hydrogenated" in the ingredient list.

*Recently, some restaurants in the U.S. have
banned trans fat from their menus, as well
as in vegetable shortening and some margarine.
Indeed, any packaged goods that contain
"partially hydrogenated vegetable oils,"
"hydrogenated vegetable oils," or
"shortening" most likely contain trans fat.
Researchers found that saturated or
trans fat increases LDL cholesterol
(the bad cholesterol) and decreases HDL
(good cholesterol), which may increase
the risk of heart disease.*

Our body fat percentage

Adipose tissue is the second most abundant substance (after water) in the human body — varying between 5% and 60%.

Males

The average male body contains 15% to 20% adipose tissue.
The average 18-year-old male contains 18% adipose tissue.
The average 65-year-old male contains 38% adipose tissue.
Ideally, healthy, lean men contain around 9% adipose tissue.
Adipose tissue content of 7% is regarded as very lean.
Adipose tissue content below 5% is regarded as unhealthy.

Females

The average female body contains 20% to 27% adipose tissue.
Ideally, healthy, lean women contain 12% to 15% adipose tissue.
Adipose tissue content below 12% is regarded as unhealthy.

Type of adipose (fat) tissue

Adipose tissue is found in the epidermis of the skin, or surrounding many organs, muscles, nerves, etc. It is made of relatively large cells that are distinguished by a thin process surrounding a large droplet of fat. The nucleus is very thin and small. Adipose tissue looks like a "honeycomb," with the cells being the walls of the chambers and the fat droplets filling the center.

We survive from meal to meal because energy is produced from stored fat as we need it. Of the average woman's body weight, 15% is fat that provides readily accessible energy. Another 4%, often referred to as "sex-specific fat" because it stores energy reserved for the demands of pregnancy and breast-feeding, is distributed primarily in the thighs, buttocks, and breasts. The average woman has enough stored fat to survive through a 60 to 90 day fast.

Fat also serves a structural purpose. Approximately 4 % of body weight is made up of fat in the organs, skeletal muscles, and central nervous systems. This fat is sometimes referred to as "essential fat" because these organs will stop functioning if it is depleted. Having too little fat is a health hazard. The risk of premature death begins to mount when body mass index (BMI) drops below 18. (BMI is calculated by multiplying weight in pounds by 700 and dividing the product by the square of height in inches.)

Adipose tissue is a specialized connective tissue that primarily acts as the main storage site for triglyceride, or fat.

In mammals, it exists in two different forms: white adipose tissue and brown adipose tissue. The body fat that human dieters are generally concerned about is stored in white adipose tissue. Excessive body fat can lead to health problems, but a certain amount of white adipose tissue is necessary for the proper functioning of the body. In addition to storing energy, the tissue, which is usually located directly below the skin, protects the body from impact-related damage to the organs and acts as a heat insulator. In addition to exercise and diet, there are a number of factors that have an apparent effect on the distribution and amount of white adipose tissue stored in a body, including gender, genetics, and race.

Brown adipose tissue derives its name from the characteristic color it gains from densely packed mitochondria and rich vascularization. Although it acts similar to white adipose tissue in some respects, it has the unique ability to generate heat. Consequently, brown adipose tissue is particularly important to small mammals in cold environments and animals in hibernation. The tissue is most prominent, however, in newborns. In fact, though brown adipose tissue comprises about 5% of the weight of human babies, it is virtually non-existent by the time adulthood is achieved.

Components of adipose tissue

It is a type of connective tissue that is specialized for the storage of neutral fats (lipids). Adipose cells have names reflecting their gross physical appearance.

▶▶ Fats (lipids) in the form of triglyceride comprise 80% to 85% of adipose tissue.

▶▶ Protein comprises 2% of adipose tissue.

▶▶ Water comprises 10% of adipose tissue.

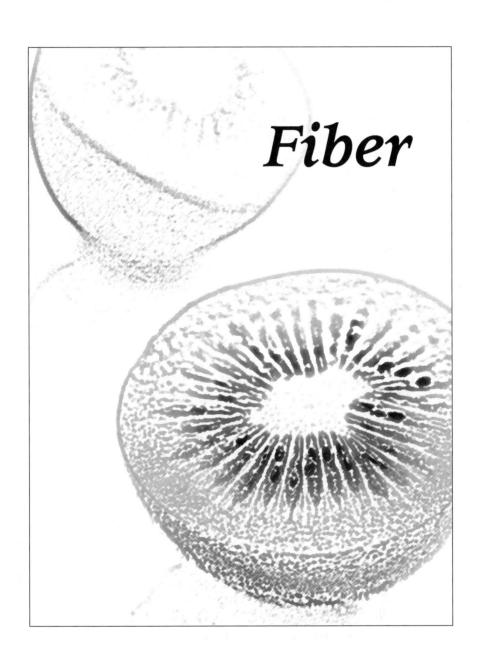

Fiber

Fiber

Fiber is one the components of food from plants that is not digestible by the human body. Even though we cannot digest it, it is still very beneficial and necessary for optimal health.

Fiber comes in two types, soluble and insoluble, depending on their ability to dissolve in water. Most foods are a mix of both types. Usually one type of fiber predominates in a food, but both are beneficial to the human body. Eating a variety of foods rich in fiber will help our bodies receive both types.

Fiber tends to expand in your stomach and give you a feeling of fullness. People who eat plenty of fiber tend to eat less quantities of food and therefore fewer calories. The result of a fiber-rich diet is that the body needs to use its fat to create energy to digest the fiber. Because fiber-rich foods are naturally packed with other nutrients, people tend to lose weight and stay slim.

A high-fiber diet causes a large, soft, bulky stool that passes through the bowel easily and quickly. Because of this action, some digestive tract disorders may also be avoided. Fiber can prevent constipation, colon polyps, and cancer of the colon. Fiber puts less strain on the colon, which helps avoid or relieve hemorrhoids.

How much and what type of fiber?

Fiber in an adult diet should aim for 20 to 35 grams daily. It's also important to remember that too much of anything, even fiber, can be bad for the body. Increase fiber intake gradually to allow time for the body to adjust. Also drink plenty of water, because fiber tends to absorb water from the body and it will need to be replaced. A good idea is to start the day with a high-fiber breakfast cereal. Include plenty of fresh vegetables during the day, and eat whole-grain products like whole wheat, rye, or brown rice bread, bulgur, brown rice, wild rice, and barley to put more fiber into your diet. Whole fresh fruit and legumes are loaded with fiber and nutrients essential for health. Try eating organically grown when making fiber choices.

Benefits of fiber

▸▸ Influences physical character of stool, a prevention and treatment of constipation.
▸▸ Modifies intestinal bacterial milieu.
▸▸ Reduces serum cholesterol (soluble fibers only).
▸▸ Binds toxins and bile salts.
▸▸ Treats diverticular disease.
▸▸ Possibly prevents hemorrhoids, varicose veins, and hiatal hernia.
▸▸ Affects absorption of carbohydrates and micro nutrients.

Role of Vitamins and Minerals in the Body

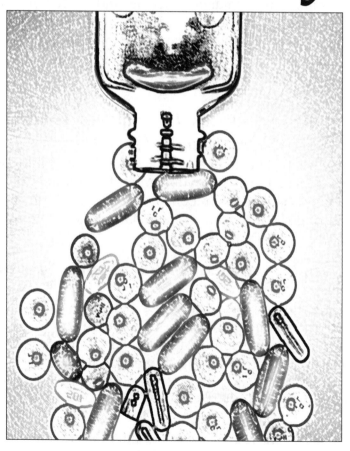

Role of vitamins and minerals in the body

Vitamins control the chemical reactions within the body that convert food into energy and living tissue. Regulating the metabolism and assisting the biochemical process that releases energy from digested food, vitamins help the body use the energy in nutrients, maintain normal body tissue, and act as a regulator. Minerals are chemical elements needed for several body functions including building strong bones, transmitting nerve signals, maintaining a normal heart beat, and are used by the body to produce necessary hormones.

There are 13 vitamins and 22 minerals we have to get from our food supply.

While only needed in small amounts, vitamins and minerals are nonetheless important because you cannot function biologically without them. According to a recent study, North Americans are lacking 72% of the nutrients they need daily. This is one of the reasons we need supplementation.

What are vitamins and what is their function?

Vitamins are tiny organic compounds that serve many different biological roles. Most help out with the biochemistry in the body, so when we become deficient in a particular vitamin, the chemical reactions in our bodies don't work as well, or at all, and we develop symptoms or become sick. Vitamins classify into two groups depending on their ability to dissolve in fat or water. They are called fat-soluble or water-soluble vitamins.

Fat-soluble vitamins are stored in the fatty tissue of the body and used when needed. Since they remain inside the body for longer periods of time, they can build up and cause problems when taken in extremely high dosages.

Water-soluble vitamins are used in the body and absorbed by the digestive system. Since they are not stored like fat-soluble vitamins, it is important to have a sufficient amount of these vitamins every day.

What are minerals?

Together with vitamins, at least 22 minerals are needed for our body functions. Some are needed in larger amounts than others and are therefore referred to as the major minerals. The others are required in smaller amounts and are called trace minerals. Major and trace minerals are equally important for the body to function.

Vitamins and minerals are sensitive compounds, meaning that they are easily destroyed, removed, or chemically altered by exposure to heat, light, or oxygen. The problem is that industrial food processing companies that process foods like white flour, refined sugar, or simply package food, often destroy or remove essential vitamins and minerals in the process. A diet high in processed foods will usually not supply enough of the vitamins and minerals we need. When we buy foods, we need to make sure that the food has not been subject to too many stresses for too long a time. Remember the earlier chart on the toxic effects of white flour?

The best preserved foods are:
▸▸ Fresh, in-season foods (especially vegetables and fruits).
▸▸ Flash frozen foods.
▸▸ Minimally processed packaged foods.
▸▸ Canned foods.

Once fresh food is in your kitchen, the way you cook it also determines the vitamin and mineral quality of the food. The best way to eat most foods is raw, with the peel intact if possible. Of

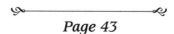

course not all foods can be eaten raw.

So alternatively, the best way to cook, which will preserve most of the vitamins and minerals, is to (1) steam, (2) broil, (3) grill, (4) stir-fry, (5) pressure cook, (6) bake, or (7) broil.

Never use the microwave for cooking. The microwave will destroy all the nutrients in some foods.

Do we need a supplement?

A multiple vitamin-mineral supplement should not replace good eating habits. Like the name suggests, it is a supplement to the foods we eat. They might not be for everyone, depending on your lifestyle factors and biochemical individuality, but most can benefit from taking a good quality and balanced supplement at the right dosage.

Many people take supplements that are not appropriate for their needs because they randomly choose a product they heard about in the news or through a friend, or just picked something from their supermarket shelf. Remember, just as your diet is best customized to your unique needs, so should your supplements be tailored to your body type and blood work. Consult with your doctor, after blood work has been done.

Note: One basic problem with the health system in the U.S. is our doctors' lack of knowledge about supplements and other nutrients. It is understandable why patients rely on other sources, so that much of what they believe is shaped by what they see, read, and hear, often from unreliable sources.

What is in a multi-vitamin?

Vitamin A

Vitamin A is a generic term for a large number of related

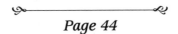

compounds. Vitamin A, a fat-soluble vitamin, plays essential roles in vision, growth, and development. The development and maintenance of healthy skin, hair, and mucous membranes; immune functions; and reproduction can be attributed to vitamin A. It also serves as a great antioxidant. Retinol (an alcohol) and retinal (an aldehyde) are often referred to as preformed vitamin A. Retinol is pure and an active vitamin A.

Another well known, synthetic form of vitamin A is tretinoin, better known as Retin-A®. Vitamin A is one of the few substances with a small enough molecular structure to penetrate the outer layers of the skin. This allows vitamin A to work at repairing the lower layers of the skin where collagen and elastin reside. It stimulates collagen and elastin, creating firmer, smoother skin. This is a good alternative for those with sensitive skin who cannot tolerate tretinoin.

Beta-carotene and other carotenoids that can be converted by the body into retinol are referred to as pro vitamin A carotenoids. Hundreds of different carotenoids are synthesized by plants, but only about 10% of them are pro vitamin A carotenoids.

The site of absorption of vitamin A is the small intestine. Good sources of vitamin A are in yellow and dark green leafy vegetables, oranges, milk fat, and organ foods such as liver and kidneys.

Health benefits of vitamin A

Vitamin A improves the stability of cell membranes by protecting the fatty acids contained in cell membranes. Vitamin A maintains and tones the epithelial cells that form the outer protective layer of skin, as well as mucous membranes.

Vitamin A deficiency may exacerbate iron deficiency anemia. Not having enough A in your system increases susceptibility to bacterial and viral diseases. A vitamin A deficiency can also cause the degeneration and atrophy of the spleen.

Here are some benefits of vitamin A:

▸▸ Used in conjunction with vitamin C, can alleviate halitosis.

▸▸ Alleviates heartburn.

▸▸ Improves the structural integrity of the mucous membrane linings of the eyes. (Note: Night blindness or poor night vision and double vision can occur as a result of vitamin A deficiency.)

▸▸ Can assist in the prevention of basal cell carcinoma, breast cancer, cervical cancer, colon cancer, and liver cancer.

▸▸ Inhibits the tumor promotion stage of lung cancer.

▸▸ Protects against pharynx cancer by strengthening the mucous membranes of the pharynx.

▸▸ Helps to prevent prostate cancer by strengthening the mucous membranes of the prostate.

▸▸ Can prevent the progress of skin cancers by stimulating normal cell differentiation.

▸▸ Stimulates various aspects of the immune system by enhancing the function of white blood cells, macrophages, neutrophils, and NK lymphocytes.

▸▸ Protects and strengthens the thymus. (Note: Supplemental vitamin A can cause the thymus to double in size.)

▸▸ Is required for the proper function of the thyroid.

▸▸ Activates retinoic acid receptors in the hippocampus, and this activation of retinoic acid receptors is essential for learning and enhances memory.

▸▸ Accelerates the healing of wounds following surgery.

▸▸ Alleviates the pancreatic insufficiency associated with cystic fibrosis.

▸▸ Alleviates and helps to prevent emphysema.

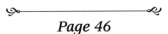

Signs of a vitamin A overdose

Toxic in large amounts, vitamin A can cause transient hydrocephalus, precocious skeletal growth, irritability, fatigue, increased intracranial pressure, anorexia, vomiting, dry and pruritic skin, loss of body hair, nystagmus, gingivitis, fissures on the tongue, hepatosplenomegaly, lymph node enlargement, slower clotting time, and increased serum alkaline phosphatase.

Vitamin D

Vitamin D is a fat-soluble vitamin. It is found in food but also can be made in your body after exposure to ultraviolet rays from the sun, an important source for D. Vitamin D exists in several forms, each with a different function. Some forms are relatively inactive in the body and have limited ability to function as a vitamin. The liver and kidney help convert vitamin D to its active hormone form as vitamin D3.

Ultraviolet (UV) rays from sunlight trigger vitamin D synthesis in the skin. It is important for individuals with limited sun exposure to include good sources of vitamin D in their diets. Such sources include fortified milk, liver, egg yolk, salmon, tuna, and sardines.

Function of vitamin D

Vitamin D is essential for normal growth and development and for the formation of strong bones and teeth. It also influences the absorption and the metabolism of phosphorus and calcium.

A diet high in oily fish prevents vitamin D deficiency.

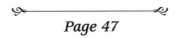

Signs of vitamin D deficiency

A lack of vitamin D can result in skeletal deformities, an increased risk for fractures, osteoporosis, osteomalacia (soft bones), rickets, muscle weakness, joint pain, and the premature closure of sutures. Serum vitamin D levels decline by up to 50% in tandem with the aging process. The deficiency of D can increase a person's chance for breast or colon cancer and has been linked with an increased risk of diabetes mellitus type 2. Fatigue can also occur as a result of vitamin D deficiency. Rheumatoid arthritis may occur as a result of vitamin D deficiency, as well as depression. Multiple sclerosis (MS) can also be considered as a danger when deficient in D, especially during puberty. Maintenance of proper vitamin D levels may delay the onset of the aging.

Health benefits of vitamin D

- Helps to prevent atherosclerosis (by stimulating the deposition of calcium in bones instead of the arteries).
- Alleviates Crohn's disease symptoms.
- Improves the absorption of vitamin A.
- Helps to prevent autoimmune diseases.
- Helps to prevent and suppress (systemic) lupus erythematous.
- Stimulates the apoptosis (programmed cell death) of some types of cancer cells (especially breast cancer cells) in D3 form.
- Helps to prevent kidney cancer.
- Inhibits the proliferation of liver cancer cells, in D3 form.
- Helps to prevent ovarian cancer.
- The calcitriol form of vitamin D helps to prevent prostate cancer (especially in men aged 57 or over).
- Enhances some functions of the immune system.
- Stimulates the activity of macrophages (cells that digest cellular debris).

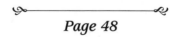

▸▸ Facilitates the production of monocytes (part of the immune system).

▸▸ Stimulates the formation and growth of the bones.

▸▸ Increases muscle strength in elderly persons.

▸▸ Helps to prevent osteoarthritis and osteoporosis.

▸▸ When consumed in conjunction with calcium, can alleviate migraines in some patients.

▸▸ Improves symptoms of MS patients.

▸▸ Is required for the production of insulin.

▸▸ Improves mood in seasonal affective disorder (SAD) patients.

It is also worth noting that vitamin D3, a form of vitamin D, increases the absorption of calcium, decreases its excretion from the kidneys, stimulates the resorption of calcium from the bones, and helps to maintain normal blood levels of calcium.

Vitamin D (after its conversion to calcitriol) helps to prevent Parkinson's disease by inhibiting the ability of 6-hydroxydopamine to exert neurotoxic effects that lead to the disease in the first place. Approximately 33% of vitamin D is converted within the liver to calcidiol. Combined with calcium, D is useful for the treatment of polycystic ovary syndrome. Combined with calcium and magnesium, it totally eliminates some cases of premenstrual syndrome (PMS).

Signs of vitamin D overdose

Toxic in large amounts, vitamin D will cause muscle weakness and loss of tone, hypocalcaemic tetany, delayed dentition, anorexia, vomiting, thirst, polyuria, fatigue, lassitude, headaches, abnormal ECG testing, shortened QT interval, and increased calcium and phosphorus. A deficiency will also decrease magnesium and increase cholesterol.

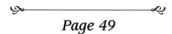

Vitamin E

Vitamin E is a fat-soluble vitamin that exists in eight different forms, four tocopherols (alpha-, beta-, gamma-, and delta-), and four tocotrienols (also alpha-, beta-, gamma-, and delta-). Each form has its own biological activity, which is the measure of potency or functional use in the body. Alpha-tocopherol is the only form of vitamin E that is actively maintained in the human body and is, therefore, the form of vitamin E found in the largest quantities in the blood and tissue. It is also a powerful biological antioxidant.

Vitamin E is absorbed in the intestine. It is found in wheat germ, vegetable oils, green leafy vegetables, egg yolks, nuts, and milk fat. As an antioxidant, it protects red blood cells from hemolysis (breaking open).

You are deficient in vitamin E if you have increased creatinuria in the urine, increased hemolysis of red blood cells, muscle weakness, decreased serum lipid levels, and steatorrhea.

Health benefits of vitamin E

▶▶ May retard the progression of the aging process.
▶▶ Facilitates the elimination of cellular waste.
▶▶ Inhibits the ability of gamma-rays to damage chromosomes and cause cell mutations.
▶▶ Exerts antioxidant effects that protect the membranes of the mitochondria from the toxic effects of free radicals generated during energy production in the mitochondria.
▶▶ Alleviates ulcerative colitis.
▶▶ Prevents gallstones and can dissolve existing gallstones.
▶▶ Alleviates the pancreatic insufficiency associated with cystic fibrosis (preferably a water-soluble form of vitamin E).
▶▶ Helps to prevent pancreatitis.
▶▶ Inhibits the cross-linking of endogenous proteins.

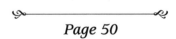

- ▶▶ Helps to prevent (diabetic) neuropathy in diabetes mellitus type 1 patients, and diabetic retinopathy.
- ▶▶ Counteracts insulin resistance in diabetes mellitus type 2.
- ▶▶ Inhibits the oxidation of LDL cholesterol (vitamin E is readily incorporated into LDL cholesterol).
- ▶▶ Inhibits the ability of homocysteine to stimulate the oxidation of LDL cholesterol.
- ▶▶ Protects the liver from oxidation damage and the toxic effects of carbon tetrachloride.
- ▶▶ Improves stamina (by enhancing respiration processes in muscle cells and heart cells).
- ▶▶ Contributes to the maintenance of normal bone growth.
- ▶▶ Improves cartilage function and improves the strength of connective tissue.
- ▶▶ Minimizes muscular atrophy during periods of immobilization.
- ▶▶ High dosages of supplemental vitamin E sometimes alleviates muscular dystrophy.
- ▶▶ Alleviates the pain associated with osteoarthritis.
- ▶▶ Contributes to the prevention of osteoporosis.
- ▶▶ Can successfully control scleroderma.

Alzheimer patients usually exhibit low blood vitamin E levels, and vitamin E helps to prevent Alzheimer's disease. Vitamin E helps to restore choline acetylase (the enzyme that generates acetylcholine) activity in Alzheimer's patients. It concentrates in the pituitary gland (the pituitary gland contains 40 micrograms of vitamin E per gram).

Signs of overdose include possible high blood pressure and increased phosphorus.

Vitamin K

Vitamin K is a fat-soluble vitamin. Chemically it is a type of quinone that plays an important role in blood clotting. The body can store fat-soluble vitamins in fatty tissue. There are two naturally occurring forms of vitamin K. Plants synthesize phylloquinone, also known as vitamin K1.

Site of absorption for this type is the upper intestine. Sources for vitamin K are liver, soybean oil, green leafy vegetables, and wheat bran. Its function is blood clotting. Many colic disease patients are found to be deficient in vitamin K. The same is true for those with Crohn's disease and those with ulcerative colitis. Vitamin K deficiency increases the risk of fractures (due to the non-production or non-activation of calcitonin). Alzheimer's disease patients generally have sub-optimal levels of vitamin K. The female body's requirement for vitamin K increases during pregnancy. It has been found that 33% of pregnant women are found to be deficient in vitamin K.

You are deficient in vitamin K if you have cutaneous purpura, ecchymosis, transient hyperprothrombinaemia, hematuria, or post-operative hemorrhaging.

Health benefits of vitamin K

▶▶ Helps to prevent atherosclerosis (by inhibiting the calcification of arteries).
▶▶ Helps prevent excessive or frequent bleeding (hemorrhage).
▶▶ Improves the health of the heart by facilitating the removal of excessive calcium from the aorta.
▶▶ Prevents stroke by inhibiting the calcification and thickening of cerebral arteries.
▶▶ Inhibits the development of many cancers including breast, colon, liver, and stomach cancer.

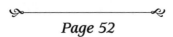

▸▸ Enhances the health of bones by activating inactive calcitonin, enabling calcitonin to transfer calcium into the bones.

▸▸ Stabilizes the synovial linings of tissues that are afflicted as a result of rheumatoid arthritis.

▸▸ Supplemental vitamin K may help to prevent and alleviate Alzheimer's disease.

▸▸ Alleviates morning sickness.

▸▸ Enhances the effectiveness of ipriflavone, when it is used to stimulate bone formation and to treat osteoporosis.

▸▸ Is involved in the synthesis of osteocalcin.

▸▸ Is essential for the production of prothrombin.

Signs of overdose include hemorrhaging, GI bleeding, epistaxis, and for synthetic vitamin K excess: kernicterus, vomiting, porphyrinuria, albuminuria, and prolonged clotting time.

Vitamin B1

Vitamin B1, also known as thiamin, helps fuel your body by converting blood sugar into energy. It keeps your mucous membranes healthy and is essential for the nervous system, cardiovascular and muscular function, the flow of electrolytes in and out of nerve and muscle cells, multiple enzyme processes, carbohydrate metabolism, and production of hydrochloric acid. Depletion of thiamin can occur as quickly as within 14 days if not enough is digested. Thiamin is not stored in large amounts in the body.

The sites of absorption are the proximal and lower duodenum. It concentrates in the kidney, liver, and brain. Sources include pork, liver, organ meats, legumes, whole-grains, wheat germ, and potatoes. B1 helps in the digestion of carbohydrates, which is essential for growth, a normal appetite, good digestion, and healthy nerves.

Signs of deficiency include central nervous system dysfunction, peripheral neuritis, nausea, vomiting, and diarrhea. Loss of appetite and constipation can occur as a result of vitamin B1 deficiency. Glaucoma patients are generally found to be deficient in vitamin B1. Many chronic fatigue syndrome (CFS) patients are found to be deficient in vitamin B1. Muscle weakness can also occur as a result of vitamin B1 deficiency. Fifty percent of the body's vitamin B1 concentrates in the muscles. Vitamin B1 deficiency increases the generation of amyloid-beta protein in the brains of Alzheimer's disease patients.

> *A deficiency of B1 has been implicated in attention deficit disorder (ADD).*

Beriberi is the classic symptom of vitamin B1 deficiency. Insomnia can also occur as a result of vitamin B1 deficiency. Numbness (especially in the feet and hands) and mouth ulcers can occur as a result of vitamin B1 deficiency, as well as a sensitive tongue or a burning sensation on the tongue.

Vitamin B1 deficiency is of particular note when it comes to the brain. It can lead to the breakdown of the blood-brain barrier, and high concentrations are found in the brain. Neuropathy can occur as a result of vitamin B1 deficiency. Poor concentration can also occur as a result of vitamin B1 deficiency, and the deficiency can actually be measured as a reduction in the thickness of the corpus callosum of the brain. Vitamin B1 deficiency can cause both delirium and depression. In addition, severe impairment of memory can occur as a result of vitamin B1 deficiency. Vitamin B1 deficiency leads to loss of neurons from the thalamus area of the brain.

Health benefits of vitamin B1

▸▸ Helps to prevent heart attacks and is useful in strengthening the heart in people who have previously suffered a heart attack.

▸▸ Is required for normal muscle tone in the heart.

▸▸ Facilitates the formation of red blood cells.

▸▸ Helps to prevent stroke.

▸▸ Alleviates hypochlorhydria (by facilitating the production of endogenous hydrochloric acid).

▸▸ Is required for the maintenance of normal muscle tone in the intestines and stomach.

▸▸ Restores vitamin B1 levels to normal via supplementation, which may be beneficial for glaucoma patients.

▸▸ Helps to prevent prostate cancer.

▸▸ Stimulates the immune system.

▸▸ Is essential for the production of energy.

▸▸ Retards the production of endogenous lactic acid (by diverting pyruvic acid into the Krebs cycle and thereby preventing its conversion to lactic acid).

▸▸ Is beneficial in the treatment of Alzheimer's disease. (It facilitates the synthesis and presynaptic release of acetylcholine and thereby improves some aspects of mental function in Alzheimer's disease patients.)

▸▸ Is required for the optimal function of the blood-brain barrier.

▸▸ Is a component of modern treatments to alleviate Down syndrome.

▸▸ Prevents and compensates for alcohol-induced damage to the hippocampus of the brain and survival of neurons in the hippocampus.

▸▸ Improves learning ability.

▸▸ Administered intraspinally, via injection, causes dramatic (but transient) improvement in the condition of multiple sclerosis

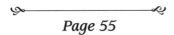

(MS) patients.

» Is an effective treatment for (the trigeminal neuralgia form of) neuralgia.

» 300 mg B1, 20 mg of B2, and 150 mg of vitamin B6 alleviates some cases of mouth ulcers.

Signs of a B1 overdose include allergies, edema, fatty liver, herpes, nervousness, sweating, tachycardia, tremors, and vascular hypertension.

Vitamin B2

Riboflavin, or vitamin B2, is a water-soluble vitamin which is involved in vital metabolic processes in the body. It is necessary for normal cell function, growth, and energy production.

Vitamin B2 is absorbed in the proximal small intestine. It also tends to concentrate in the retina. Its sources include milk and other dairy, organ meats, green leafy vegetables, and eggs.

It is essential for growth. Coenzymes form flavin adenine dinucleotide (FAD), a group of endogenous flavins that are a component of many flavoproteins. Flavin mononucleotide is an endogenous flavin and is an enzyme in the body which helps tissues to respire.

Signs of deficiency include burning

What you need to know about Ascorbic Acid

Ascorbic acid is the simplest, most readily available form of Vitamin C. However, since ascorbic acid is water soluble, the body will always have problems storing it. While the absorption of water soluble vitamin C is quite quick, its penetration into cells is limited. Unlike Vitamin E, a fat soluble vitamin, vitamin C is not stored in the body. This makes ascorbyl palmitate, a fat-soluble form of Vitamin C supplementation very attractive.

There is a chemical process in which Vitamin C can be made in a lab and it can even legally be labeled as Vitamin C, which is very misleading to consumers. This processed type of C is missing 80% of what constitutes food grade Vitamin C. Even worse, researchers from the University of California reported in 2000 that people who took 500 mgs of ascorbic acid had a 2.5 times faster progression of hardening of the arteries than people who took no supplement at all.

A better way to take Vitamin C

Ascorbyl palmitate is an ester formed from ascorbic acid and palmitic acid creating a fat-soluble form of vitamin C. Unlike ascorbic acid, which is water-soluble, ascorbyl palmitate is not. Consequently ascorbyl palminate can be stored in cell membranes until it is required by the body. Many people think vitamin C (ascorbyl palminate) is only used for immune support, but it has many other important functions. A major role of vitamin C is in manufacturing collagen, a protein that forms the basis of connective tissue - the most abundant tissue in the body. Ascorbyl palmitate is an effective free radical-scavenging antioxidant which promotes skin health and vitality. Ascorbyl palmitate, working at the cell membrane, has been shown to provide antioxidant action comparable, or even greater than, that of vitamin E. It also acts synergistically with vitamin E, helping to regenerate the vitamin E radical on a constant basis..

of the eyes, dim vision, and phobia. In the skin, vitamin B2 deficiency shows up as angular stomatitis, chelosis, or seborrheic dermatitis. Magenta tongue is another sign of a lack of B2, as is glossitis (red, sore, or smooth tongue, sore tip, or enlarged taste buds). Many chronic fatigue syndrome patients are found to be deficient in vitamin B2. Thyroid malfunction can occur from a lack of vitamin B2, as can carpal tunnel syndrome and depression. Tingling or a burning sensation in the feet or hands are other deficiency symptoms. Angular stomatosis (cracks in the corner of the mouth) can occur. Cracked lips can also occur as a result of vitamin B2 deficiency.

People who exercise regularly have a higher daily requirement for vitamin B2 than those who are sedentary, due to vitamin B2's ability to protect the body's energy manufacturing processes from oxidative damage.

Vitamin B2 should not be used by pre-existing cataract patients as some evidence suggests that supplemental vitamin B2 may exacerbate existing cataracts.

Health benefits of vitamin B2

- ▸▸ Facilitates the production of red blood cells.
- ▸▸ Enhances cell respiration by facilitating the ability of cells to efficiently utilize oxygen, and alleviates sickle cell anemia.
- ▸▸ Is useful in the treatment of gastric ulcers and duodenal ulcers.
- ▸▸ Alleviates tearing of the eyes.
- ▸▸ Is essential for the production of antibodies.
- ▸▸ Helps to prevent colon cancer and esophagus cancer.
- ▸▸ Helps to prevent prostate cancer (in part by inhibiting the five-alpha reductase enzyme that catalyzes the conversion of testosterone to dihydrotestosterone).
- ▸▸ Combined with vitamin B12, it reduces the risk of alcohol (ethanol) induced cirrhosis.
- ▸▸ Alleviates fatigue.
- ▸▸ Facilitates the formation of collagen in damaged connective tissues that are affected by carpal tunnel syndrome.
- ▸▸ Is an adjunct in the treatment of Alzheimer's disease (when combined with supplemental taurine and zinc).
- ▸▸ 400 mg per day helps to prevent migraines by improving the efficiency with which energy is produced by the mitochondria. (Reduction in the production of energy by the mitochondria is proposed as an underlying cause of migraine.)
- ▸▸ Alleviates eczema.
- ▸▸ Heals rosacea when rosacea is caused by vitamin B2 deficiency.

There are no signs of overdose as vitamin B2 is essentially non-toxic.

Vitamin B3 (niacin, nicotinic acid, nicotinamide, niacinamide)

Vitamin B3, or niacin, is a water-soluble vitamin whose derivatives, such as NADH, play essential roles in energy metabolism in the living cell. Like all the B-complex vitamins, it is important for converting calories from protein, fat, and carbohydrates into energy. But it also helps the digestive system function and promotes a normal appetite, healthy skin, and nerves. Niacin is required for cell respiration, proper circulation, healthy skin, functioning of the nervous system, and normal secretion of bile and stomach fluids. It is used in the synthesis of sex hormones.

Vitamin B3 is absorbed in the intestine. Its sources are fish, liver, meat, poultry, many grains, eggs, peanuts, milk, and legumes.

This B acts in the metabolism of carbohydrates and amino acids. It is involved in glycolysis, fat synthesis, and tissue respiration.

Signs of deficiency include achlorhydria, dermatitis, retarded growth, increased pulse rate, increased respiratory rate, loss of memory, pigmentation, and diarrhea.

Signs of overdose include low blood pressure, burning, itching skin, fatty liver, peripheral vasodilation, decreased serum cholesterol, stimulated central nervous system, and increased cerebral blood flow.

Health benefits of all forms of vitamin B3

- ▶ The niacinamide form of vitamin B3 is an effective adjunct therapy for the early treatment of stroke.
- ▶ Alleviates hypochlorhydria (by stimulating the production of hydrochloric acid).
- ▶ In high doses can alleviate some cases of tinnitus.

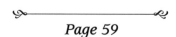

➨ Applied topically may enhance hair re-growth in persons afflicted with male pattern baldness.

➨ Is involved in the metabolism of carbohydrates to energy.

➨ The niacinamide form of vitamin B3 helps to prevent the onset of diabetes mellitus type 1 (by protecting the beta cells of the islets of Langerhans from destruction).

➨ Niacinamide form stabilizes blood sugar levels in diabetes mellitus type 2 patients.

➨ Is essential for the body's production of energy (due to its role in the manufacture of adenosine triphosphate).

➨ Is involved in the body's hydrogen transfer system (as an essential component of the coenzymes nicotinamide adenine dinucleotide and nicotinamide adenine dinucleotide phosphate).

➨ Alleviates hypoglycemia.

➨ Lowers low density lipoprotein (LDL) levels.

Vitamin B6

Vitamin B6 is a water-soluble vitamin that exists in three major chemical forms: pyridoxine, pyridoxal, and pyridoxamine. It performs a wide variety of functions in your body and is essential for your good health. For example, vitamin B6 is needed for more than 100 enzymes involved in protein metabolism. It is also essential for red blood cell metabolism. The nervous and immune systems need vitamin B6 to function efficiently, and it is also needed for the conversion of tryptophan (an amino acid) to niacin (vitamin B3). It helps maintain the health of lymphoid organs (thymus, spleen, and lymph nodes) that make the body's white blood cells.

Human bodies need vitamin B6 to make hemoglobin to carry oxygen to the tissues. Vitamin B6 also helps increase the amount of oxygen carried by hemoglobin. Vitamin B6 deficiency can cause anemia, which is similar to iron deficiency anemia. Vitamin B6 also helps maintain body blood glucose (sugar) within a normal range. It aids in synthesis and breakdown of amino acids, which is essential in conversion of tryptophan to niacin. B6 aids in the synthesis of unsaturated fatty acids from essential fatty acids, necessary for normal growth.

Vitamin B6 is absorbed by the upper small intestine. It is found in pork, glandular meats, cereal bran and germ, milk, egg yolk, oatmeal, and legumes. It is also made by intestinal bacteria.

Signs of deficiency include anemia, peripheral neuritis, and cutaneous. Most celiac disease patients are found to be deficient in vitamin B6, as are most diabetes mellitus patients. Hepatitis can occur as a result of vitamin B6 deficiency and hepatitis significantly increases the body's vitamin B6 requirements. Muscle weakness and pain can also occur as a result of vitamin B6 deficiency. Insufficient vitamin B6 can result in insomnia and irritability. Migraines can also occur as a result of vitamin B6 deficiency, and there may be an increased risk of multiple sclerosis. Vitamin B6 deficiency can cause neuropathy.

Signs of overdose are nominal as B6 has a limited toxicity. However, dosages of vitamin B6 in excess of 500 mg per day can cause sensory neuropathy. This effect occurs with excess vitamin B6 due to conversion of the stimulatory neurotransmitter — glutamic acid — to the inhibitory neurotransmitter — gamma amino-butyric acid. Dosages of supplemental vitamin B6 above 2,000 mg per day impair the sense of pain, temperature, and touch.

Health benefits of vitamin B6

▶ Helps to prevent atherosclerosis (by helping to break down atherosclerotic plaque and by preventing the build-up of homocysteine).
▶ Helps to prevent abnormal blood clotting.
▶ Helps to prevent ischemic heart disease.

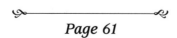

▸▸ Lowers blood pressure in hypertension patients (by influencing the nervous system's participation in the control of blood pressure).

▸▸ Helps to prevent intermittent claudication (by helping to lower elevated homocysteine levels).

▸▸ Reduces the severity of Raynaud's disease.

▸▸ Facilitates the production of red blood cells (due to its involvement in the production of hemoglobin).

▸▸ Facilitates the removal of the toxic substances that cause body odor.

▸▸ Alleviates hypochlorhydria (by stimulating the endogenous production of hydrochloric acid).

▸▸ Prevents the formation of kidney stones that are caused by hyperoxaluria (due to its role in the metabolism of oxalic acid).

▸▸ Facilitates the excretion of urine (due to its influence on the body's sodium/potassium balance).

▸▸ Helps prevent the HIV virus from infecting T-lymphocytes by blocking the CD4 receptors located on T-lymphocytes.

▸▸ Alleviates allergies (by functioning as a cofactor for the histaminase enzyme that degrades excessive histamine).

▸▸ Retards the growth of some forms of cancer including bladder, colon, liver, lung, and pancreatic.

▸▸ Is essential for the production and secretion of antibodies.

▸▸ Is essential for the production of B-lymphocytes and T-lymphocytes.

▸▸ Increases the number of helper T-cells.

▸▸ Improves the ability of neutrophils to function as phagocytes.

▸▸ Retards the oxidation of LDL cholesterol and lowers total serum LDL cholesterol levels.

▸▸ Is useful for the treatment of chronic fatigue syndrome.

▸▸ Inhibits the cross-linking (glycosylation) of endogenous proteins.

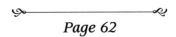

▸ Is useful for the treatment of fibrocystic breast disease (especially in women who experience pre-menstrual syndrome in conjunction with the disease).

▸ Shrinks the synovial membranes that line the surface of the joints, thereby alleviating pain in the joints and restoring mobility to the joints.

▸ Reduces the size and inflammation of Hebderden's nodes in osteoarthritis patients.

▸ Alleviates and controls rheumatism (by shrinking the synovial membranes that line the surface of the joints, thereby alleviating pain and restoring mobility).

▸ Improves the mental function of Alzheimer's disease patients (by inhibiting the acetylcholinesterase enzyme that is over-active in these patients).

▸ Facilitates the production of serotonin in attention deficit disorder (ADD) patients. (Serotonin is often depleted in ADD patients.)

▸ 200 mg taken at bedtime improves the ability to recall dreams and also increases their intensity and color. (Effects are usually noticeable three nights after commencing this regime.)

▸ Improves long-term memory in elderly persons.

▸ Facilitates the development and health of the myelin sheaths that cover the nerves, which allows them to conduct nerve impulses.

▸ Increases the production of dopamine.

▸ 100 mg of vitamin B6 per day results in improved bladder control, steadier gait, decreased cramps, trembling, and rigidity in Parkinson's disease patients. (Note: Parkinson's disease patients should not use supplemental vitamin B6 in conjunction with supplemental L-dopa, which vitamin B6 inactivates in the intestines.)

Vitamin B9

Folic acid and folate (the anion form) are forms of the water-soluble vitamin B9. These occur naturally in food and can also be taken as supplements. Folate is necessary for the development of the neural tube that encloses the spinal cord.

It is absorbed in the jejunum and small intestine. Vitamin B9 is found in wheat, eggs, fish, dry beans, lentils, asparagus, green leafy vegetables, organ meats, lean beef, broccoli, and yeast. It is also made in the intestinal tract.

B9 is essential for biosynthesis of nucleic acids, which are necessary for normal maturation of red blood cells.

Signs of deficiency include megaloblastic anemia, central nervous system changes, glottises, hepatomegaly, hyperpigmentation, thrombocytopenia, intestinal disturbances, leukopenia, and sprue. Many chronic fatigue syndrome (CFS) patients are found to be deficient in folic acid, as are patients with celiac disease and Crohn's disease. Fatigue can occur as a result of folic acid deficiency.

There are no signs of overdose, as no toxicity has ever been reported.

Health benefits of folic acid

▶▶ Helps to protect against intestinal parasites.
▶▶ Reduces the risk of colon cancer in ulcerative colitis patients. (Ulcerative colitis patients generally have a significantly increased risk of colon cancer.)
▶▶ At least 400 mcg per day consumed by women during pregnancy helps to prevent most neural tube defects (especially spina bifida).
▶▶ Prevents some forms of cancer including breast, cervical, colon, esophageal, lung, ovarian, pancreatic, stomach, and uterus cancer.

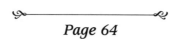

Vitamin B12

Vitamin B12 (cobalamin) is a water-soluble vitamin. In contrast to other water-soluble vitamins, it is not excreted quickly in the urine, but rather accumulates and is stored in the liver, kidney, and other body tissues. As a result, a vitamin B12 deficiency may not manifest itself until after five or six years of a diet supplying inadequate amounts. Vitamin B12 functions as a methyl donor and works with folic acid in the synthesis of DNA and red blood cells and is vitally important in maintaining the health of the insulation sheath (myelin sheath) that surrounds nerve cells. The classical vitamin B12 deficiency disease is pernicious anemia, a serious disease characterized by large, immature red blood cells. It is now clear that a vitamin B12 deficiency can have serious consequences long before anemia is evident.

Vitamin B12 is absorbed in the terminal ileum. It is found in animal products, milk, eggs only, and fish.

B12 is involved in the metabolism of single-carbon fragments, essential for biosynthesis of nucleic acids and nucleoproteins. It is also involved with folate metabolism. B12's role in the metabolism of nervous tissue is related to growth. The body's ability to absorb dietary vitamin B12 declines as we age. Daily supplements of 500 to 1,000 micrograms are recommended in order to counteract this impaired absorption in persons over the age of 60.

Signs of deficiency include megaloblastic/pernicious anemia, gastrointestinal tract changes, nerve damage, peripheral neuropathy, diminished sense of position and vibration, poor growth, sore-smooth tongue, splenomegaly, and thrombocytopenia. Nervousness is one of the initial symptoms of vitamin B12 deficiency, as well as numbness of the hands and feet, and dry mouth. Patients with celiac disease are found to be deficient in vitamin B12. B12 deficiency is common in Crohn's disease patients; however, this does not imply that vitamin B12 alleviates Crohn's disease. It does imply that Crohn's disease patients may need to supplement with vitamin B12 (administered by a physician via injection) in order to avoid B12 deficiency. The sole absorption site for vitamin B12 is in the ileum, the same site that is most commonly impaired by Crohn's disease.

Vitamin B12 deficiency contributes to hypochlorhydria. It can lead to age-related hearing loss. Some cases of tinnitus are attributable to vitamin B12 deficiency (47% of tinnitus patients exhibit vitamin B12 deficiency). Vitamin B12 is beneficial due to its ability to enhance the conduction of nerve impulses relating to hearing. Vitamin B12 deficiency impairs the function of the optic nerve. Chronic fatigue syndrome (CFS) patients generally have abnormally low vitamin B12 levels and supplemental vitamin B12 (2.5 to 5 mg per day administered via injection or 5 to 10 mg administered orally) may be useful for treatment. Depression can occur as a result of vitamin B12 deficiency. During pregnancy, a lack of vitamin B12 can result in impaired development of myelin sheaths in offspring. Tobacco smokers are often found to be deficient in vitamin B12. A deficiency can also cause abnormally heavy bleeding during menstruation.

Signs of overdose include polycythemia.

Health benefits of vitamin B12

▶▶ Helps to prevent atherosclerosis and heart attacks (primarily by reducing toxic levels of homocysteine).
▶▶ Is essential for the formation of red blood cells and integrity of cell membranes.
▶▶ Is essential for the production of all epithelial cells.
▶▶ The methylcobalamin form of B12 may help to prevent glaucoma (by inhibiting the toxicity of glutamic acid, a suspected cause of glaucoma; and by preserving myelin).

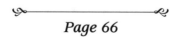

▸▸ 1 to 2 mg per day improves the condition of viral hepatitis patients.

▸▸ Helps to prevent breast cancer.

▸▸ Optimizes the ratios of the various types of white blood cells and raises suppressed white blood cell (helper T-cells, lymphocytes, NK lymphocytes) counts.

▸▸ Improves the metabolism of carbohydrates and dietary fats.

▸▸ Combined with vitamin B2, reduces the risk of alcohol (ethanol)-induced cirrhosis.

▸▸ May be useful for the treatment of hepatitis C.

▸▸ Administered intramuscularly, alleviates the pain associated with backache.

▸▸ May be useful for the treatment of fibromyalgia.

▸▸ In the methylcobalamin form, retards the nerve degeneration that occurs in muscular dystrophy patients.

▸▸ Has been linked to the development of Alzheimer's disease.

▸▸ Administered concurrently with folic acid, alleviates anxiety.

▸▸ In the methylcobalamin form, accelerates recovery from Bell's palsy.

▸▸ Alleviates delayed sleep phase disorder.

▸▸ Improves some aspects (frontal lobe function and language skills) of dementia.

▸▸ 1 mg consumed immediately prior to falling asleep often (in approximately 50% of people) causes vivid, brightly colored dreams.

▸▸ Supplementation with massive doses of vitamin B12 (oral administration of 60 mg of the methylcobalamin form) improves visual and brainstem auditory-evoked nerve potentials by up to 30% in MS patients, but does not improve motor function.

▸▸ Facilitates the production of ribonucleic acid within neurons, and the methylcobalamin form of vitamin B12 helps to prevent the damage to neurons caused by exposure to

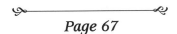

excessive levels of glutamic acid.

▸▸ In methylcobalamin form, facilitates the regeneration of damaged axons.

▸▸ The (active coenzyme) adenosylcobalamin or methylcobalamin forms of vitamin B12 help to maintain the correct fatty acid environment in the myelin sheaths that surround neurons.

▸▸ Facilitates the incorporation of the correct amino acids (leucine) into Schwann cells.

▸▸ Helps to alleviate the pain associated with the (post herpetic) neuralgia associated with shingles.

▸▸ Administered concurrently with folic acid, helps to control panic disorder.

▸▸ Administered via intramuscular injection, reduces the pain associated with sciatica.

▸▸ Alleviates mouth ulcers.

▸▸ 1 - 6 mg per day increases sperm counts in men afflicted with male infertility.

▸▸ 1 mg per day alleviates chronic dermatitis and eczema.

Vitamin B5

Pantothenic acid, or vitamin B5, is one of eight water-soluble B vitamins. All B vitamins help the body to convert carbohydrates into glucose, which turns to energy. These B vitamins, often referred to as B complex vitamins, are essential in the breakdown of fats and protein. B complex vitamins also play an important role in maintaining muscle tone in the gastrointestinal tract and promoting the health of the nervous system, skin, hair, eyes, mouth, and liver.

Pantothenic acid is found throughout living cells in the form of coenzyme A (CoA), a vital coenzyme in numerous chemical reactions. CoA is required for chemical reactions that generate energy from food (fat, carbohydrates, and proteins). The synthesis of essential fats, cholesterol, and steroid hormones requires CoA, as does the synthesis of the neurotransmitter, acetylcholine, and the hormone melatonin. Heme, a component of hemoglobin, requires a CoA-containing compound for its synthesis.

Pantothenic acid is absorbed in the intestines. It is present in all plant and animal foods. The best sources are kidney, liver, salmon, and yeast.

It is essential in the intermediary metabolism of carbohydrate, fat, and protein. As part of CoA, panthothnic acid functions in the synthesis and breakdown of many vital body compounds, and CoA is needed for metabolism of a number of drugs and toxins by the liver.

Signs of deficiency include cardiovascular changes, depression, digestive disorders, greater susceptibility to infection, neuromotor disturbances, and physical weakness. Fatigue is the most common symptom of vitamin B5 deficiency. Hypoglycemia can also occur as a result of a lack of vitamin B5. Impaired adrenal gland function, including impaired production of adrenal hormones, can occur as a result of B5 deficiency, as can adrenal cortex failure. Hypochlorhydria (insufficient production of hydrochloric acid) and depression can also occur.

There is also an increased risk of upper respiratory tract infections.

Pantothenic acid is essentially non-toxic, so you cannot be overdosed.

Health benefits of pantothenic acid

- ▶▶ Enhances the production of red blood cells.
- ▶▶ Increases the body's production of antibodies.
- ▶▶ Helps to prevent bacterial and viral infections by stimulating the production of antibodies.
- ▶▶ In pantethine form, activates NK lymphocytes.

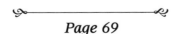

▸▸ Improves athletic performance due to its role in the production of energy.

▸▸ Reduces the synthesis of endogenous cholesterol from mevalonic acid.

▸▸ Above 500 mg per day, increases HDL and lowers LDL cholesterol levels.

▸▸ Essential for the conversion of fats, carbohydrates, and proteins into energy due to its role as a precursor for the production of adenosine triphosphate and acetyl coenzyme A.

▸▸ In pantethine form, alleviates hepatitis A.

▸▸ In pantethine form, inhibits the ability of alcohol (ethanol) and carbon tetrachloride to damage the liver.

▸▸ In pantethine form, inhibits the ability of Ibuprofen to destroy liver cells.

▸▸ Facilitates weight loss in persons afflicted with obesity (by facilitating the processes of thermogenesis, beta-oxidation, and peristalsis).

▸▸ Markedly reduces joint pain and joint stiffness associated with osteoarthritis.

Biotin (vitamin H)

Biotin, a member of the B-vitamin family, is an essential nutrient in human nutrition. It is involved in the biosynthesis of fatty acids, gluconeogenesis, energy production, the metabolism of the branched chain amino acids (L-leucine, L-isoleucine, L-valine), and the de novo synthesis of purine nucleotides. Biotin is a water-soluble vitamin produced in the body by certain types of intestinal bacteria and obtained from food.

Biotin is absorbed in the upper small intestine. It can be found in liver, mushrooms, peanuts, yeast, milk, meat, egg yolk, vegetables, bananas, grapefruit, tomato, watermelon, and strawberries. It is also made in the intestinal tract.

Biotin is an essential component of enzymes and involved in the synthesis and breakdown of fatty acids and amino acids.

Signs of deficiency include anorexia, anemia, and dermatitis. Not enough biotin can result in non-pruritic scalp, cheeks, neck, groin, and gluteal regions. Nausea and vomiting can occur as a result of biotin deficiency. It can cause atrophy (shrinkage) of the thymus gland, anorexia nervosa, depression, headaches, and hair loss. Dry skin or flaky skin can also occur as a result of biotin deficiency. The most common cause of seborrheic dermatitis is biotin deficiency.

Biotin is essentially non-toxic so cannot be overdosed.

Health benefits of biotin

- ▸ Improves the function of the digestive system by enhancing the actions of those digestive enzymes that are present in pancreatic juice secreted by the pancreas.
- ▸ Helps to prevent and suppress infection by candida albicans (primarily by preventing candida albicans from converting to its rhizoid form).
- ▸ Required for the production of lymphocytes.
- ▸ Helps to regulate blood sugar levels, which alleviates diabetes mellitus.
- ▸ Helps to prevent and treat neuropathy in diabetes mellitus patients.
- ▸ Reduces insulin resistance.
- ▸ Enhances the function of the liver.
- ▸ Alleviates some cases of muscle pain and muscle weakness.
- ▸ In large doses, helps to prevent and treat diabetic neuropathy in diabetes mellitus patients.
- ▸ May delay the onset of gray hair and may retard the further progression of gray hair.

▸▸ Alleviates brittle nails.

▸▸ Normalizes secretions of the sebaceous glands.

▸▸ Facilitates the incorporation of amino acids into endogenous proteins.

▸▸ Involved in the metabolism of carbohydrates.

▸▸ Increases the activity of glucokinase.

▸▸ Improves insulin sensitivity (i.e. it reduces insulin resistance).

▸▸ Involved in the metabolism of dietary fats.

▸▸ Involved in the endogenous synthesis of fatty acids.

▸▸ Facilitates the synthesis of endogenous nucleic acids.

▸▸ Facilitates the synthesis and breakdown of purines.

▸▸ Is a cofactor for the synthesis of endogenous pyrimidines (raw materials for nucleotides).

▸▸ Facilitates the incorporation of amino acids into endogenous proteins.

▸▸ Enhances the function of vitamins B2, B3, B6, B12, and vitamin A.

▸▸ Improves the absorption of vitamin C.

Vitamin C

Vitamin C, also known as ascorbic acid, is a water-soluble vitamin. Unlike most mammals, humans do not have the ability to make their own vitamin C. Therefore, we must obtain vitamin C through our diet. Vitamin C is also a highly effective antioxidant. Vitamin C is required for the synthesis of collagen and is an important structural component of blood vessels, tendons, ligaments, and bone. Vitamin C also plays an important role in the synthesis of the neurotransmitter, norepinephrine. Neurotransmitters are critical to brain function and are known to affect mood. In addition, vitamin C is required for the synthesis of carnitine, a small molecule that is essential for the transport of fat to cellular organelles called mitochondria, for conversion to energy.

Site of absorption is the small intestine. Vitamin C concentrates in the female ovaries and in the testes of the male testicles. It is found in citrus fruit, tomatoes, melons, peppers, greens, raw cabbage, guava, strawberries, pineapples, and potatoes.

Vitamin C maintains the intracellular cement substance with the preservation of capillary integrity. It is a co-substrate in hydroxylations requiring molecular oxygen. Important in immune responses, wound healing, and allergic reactions, vitamin C also increases absorption of iron and antioxidants.

Signs of deficiency include poor wound healing and scurvy. Excessive bleeding can occur as a result of severe vitamin C deficiency (due to fragile capillaries), and excessive bleeding is a primary symptom of scurvy. Vitamin C deficiency can cause hemorrhoids. The female body's requirement for vitamin C increases during pregnancy. Vitamin C deficiency is common in Crohn's disease patients; however, this does not imply that vitamin C alleviates Crohn's disease. These patients may need to supplement with vitamin C in order to avoid a deficiency.

Excess amounts of vitamin C do not produce a hypervitaminosis, but they are linked to oxalate stones and gout in susceptible people.

Health benefits of vitamin C

▸▸ Alleviates the methemoglobinemia form of anemia by converting toxic methemoglobin back to hemoglobin.
▸▸ Alleviates the iron deficiency form of anemia by facilitating iron absorption.
▸▸ Prevents excessive post-surgery bleeding.

▶ Helps to prevent abnormal blood clotting by inhibiting the production of prostaglandin E2. (In one study the daily administration of 2,000 mg of vitamin C prevented the formation of new blood clots and caused existing blood clots to disappear.)
▶ Helps to prevent atherosclerosis in tobacco smokers by improving the function of the endothelium.
▶ Strengthens the arteries by enhancing the incorporation of collagen into the walls of the arteries.
▶ Alleviates hemorrhoids by strengthening the blood vessels.
▶ Reduces the severity of Raynaud's disease.
▶ Inhibits the manufacture of excessive apoprotein, which is strongly implicated in various forms of cardiovascular diseases.
▶ Reduces systolic blood pressure in hypertension patients.
▶ Helps to prevent ischemic heart disease.
▶ Helps to increase sexual desire by facilitating the production of sexual steroid hormones.
▶ Helps to prevent preeclampsia in women.
▶ Alleviates male infertility by improving sperm motility and quality.
▶ Improves sperm quality, motility, and viability in male tobacco smokers and protects the sperm from the genetic damage that can cause hereditary diseases in offspring.
▶ Alleviates constipation.
▶ Reduces the incidence of gallbladder disease and helps to prevent gallstones.
▶ Helps to prevent and treat chronic pancreatitis due to the antioxidant properties of vitamin C.

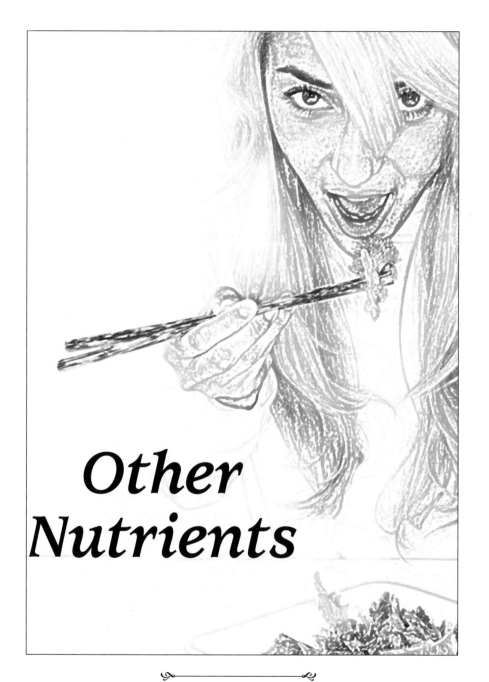

Other Nutrients

Minerals

Calcium

Calcium, the most abundant mineral in the human body, has several important functions. More than 99% of total body calcium is stored in the bones and teeth, where it functions to support their structure. The remaining 1% is found throughout the body in blood, muscle, and the fluid between cells. Calcium is needed for muscle contraction, blood vessel contraction and expansion, the secretion of hormones and enzymes, and for sending messages through the nervous system. A constant level of calcium is maintained in body fluid and tissues so that these vital body processes function efficiently.

Osteoclasts, the components of bone cells, begin the process of rebuilding bone by dissolving or re-absorbing bone. Bone-forming cells called osteoblasts then synthesize new bone to replace the bone that was re-absorbed. During normal growth, bone formation exceeds bone resorption. Osteoporosis may result when bone resorption exceeds formation. An average of 700 mg of calcium moves into and out of the human body's bones each day.

Calcium is mainly absorbed in the duodenum and jejunum. Its sources include milk, yogurt, cheese, green leafy vegetables, nuts, grains, beans, canned salmon, sardines, oysters, and tofu.

Calcium is needed to build and maintain bones and teeth. It also serves in the transport function of cell membranes, but acting as a membrane stabilizer. Calcium is required in nerve transmission and regulation of your heartbeat. This vital mineral influences transmission of ions across cell membranes, the release of neurotransmitters at synaptic junctions, the function of protein hormones, and the release or activation of intracellular and extracellular enzymes. The proper balance of calcium, sodium potassium, and magnesium maintains muscle tone and controls nerve irritability. Ionized calcium initiates the formation of a blood clot by stimulating the release of thromboplastin from the blood platelets. Calcium is also a necessary co-factor in the conversion of prothrombin to thrombin, which aids in the polymerization of fibrinogen to fibrin.

Osteoporosis (brittle bones) is a sure sign of a calcium deficiency, as are tetany and hypertension.

Signs of a calcium overdose include a bitter taste, lethargy, inability to sleep, coma, anorexia, constipation, subcutaneous fat necrosis, renal calcification, and kidney stones.

Calcium deficiency causes loss of bone calcium, which can result in bone pain and osteoporosis. Osteomalacia can also occur. In fact, many bone ailments can occur as a result of calcium deficiency. Rickets can occur due to insufficient calcium, although rickets usually occur as a result of a vitamin D deficiency. Abnormalities in calcium homeostasis appear to be a primary factor in the pathogenesis of hypertension. Post-menopausal women afflicted with depression are often deficient in calcium, and supplemental calcium may alleviate this problem not only in post-menopausal women, but in elderly patients as well. A herpes simplex outbreak can be a symptom of calcium deficiency. Brittle nails are also a symptom. Calcium intake of over 3,000 mg per day is detrimental to the brain.

Health benefits of calcium

▶▶ Enhances the function of the adrenal glands.

▶▶ Enhances growth of the bones.

▶▶ Helps to prevent fractures.

▶▶ 800 to 1,500 mg of calcium per day significantly increases bone mass in post-menopausal women.

▶▶ Enhances the blood clotting or coagulation process.

▶▶ Activates prothrombin, which converts fibrinogen to fibrin.

▶▶ Can regulate blood pH balance.

▶▶ Up to 1,500 mg per day lowers blood pressure in many hypertension patients.

▶▶ At optimal levels, acts as its own calcium channel blocker, controlling its own influx across the cell membrane.

▶▶ Normalizes heart rhythm in arrhythmia patients, as calcium allows the heart muscles to contract.

▶▶ Facilitates the normal process of apoptosis, which helps to destroy some types of cancer cells.

▶▶ Improves the permeability of cell membranes.

▶▶ Prevents bile acids from becoming carcinogenic by binding to them and enhancing their elimination from the body.

▶▶ Helps to prevent constipation.

▶▶ Helps to prevent kidney stones, except in people with hypercalciuria (abnormally high excretion of calcium via the urine, in which case additional calcium increases the risk of kidney stones).

▶▶ Involved in the optimal function of the kidneys.

▶▶ May reduce the incidence of colon cancer by forming insoluble compounds with some mild carcinogens produced within the body, including bile acids.

▶▶ Binds to and prevents fatty acids from becoming carcinogenic, which contributes to calcium's ability to reduce the incidence of colon cancer.

▸▸ Required for the production of adenosine triphosphate.

▸▸ Increases HDL and lowers LDL cholesterol levels.

▸▸ Facilitates weight loss in persons afflicted with obesity.

▸▸ Allows muscles to contract.

▸▸ Sedates the central nervous system.

▸▸ When consumed in conjunction with vitamin D, alleviates migraines in some patients.

▸▸ Used in conjunction with magnesium and vitamin D, reduces the severity of multiple sclerosis.

▸▸ Involved in the transmission of nerve impulses.

▸▸ The ovaries require calcium for the production of estrogens.

▸▸ Combined with vitamin D, is useful for the treatment of polycystic ovary syndrome.

Phosphorus

Phosphorus is an essential mineral that is required by every cell in the body for normal function. The majority of the phosphorus in the body is found as phosphate (PO_4). Approximately 85% of the body's phosphorus is found in bone in the form of a calcium phosphate salt called hydroxyapatite. Phospholipids (i.e. phosphatidylcholine) are major structural components of cell membranes. All energy production and storage are dependent on phosphorylated compounds, such as adenosine triphosphate (ATP) and creatine phosphate. Nucleic acids (DNA and RNA), responsible for the storage and transmission of genetic information, are long chains of phosphate-containing molecules. A number of enzymes, hormones, and cell-signaling molecules depend on phosphorylation for their activation. Phosphorus also helps to maintain normal acid-base balance (pH) in its role as one of the body's most important buffers.

Phosphorus is absorbed in the small intestine. It is found in cheese, egg yolk, milk, meat, fish, poultry, whole-grain cereals,

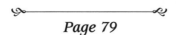

legumes, and nuts.

Its main structural role is in bones and teeth, but it is also an essential component of nucleic acids and phospholipids, which are key components in the structure of cell membranes.

Signs of deficiency include neuromuscular weakness, skeletal weakness, and hematological and renal abnormalities, which occur due to decreased ATP.

Signs of overdose are not common but may include hypocalcemia, with possible resulting tetany.

Health benefits of phosphorus

▶▶ In the form of phosphates such as calcium phosphate, potassium phosphate, or sodium phosphate, can increase the ability of the blood to transport oxygen to the muscles and increases maximum oxygen uptake.

▶▶ Helps to prevent decreases in plasma triiodothyronine (T3) levels.

▶▶ Provides the phosphate in the adenosine diphosphate molecule, the adenosine monophosphate molecule, the adenosine triphosphate molecule, and the creatine phosphate molecule.

▶▶ Facilitates the transportation of fatty acids through the body.

▶▶ Is a component of phospholipids and sphingolipids.

▶▶ Is an essential cofactor for the conversion of L-dopa to dopamine.

▶▶ Is an essential component of the nucleotides that form polynucleotides such as deoxyribonucleic acid (DNA) and ribonucleic acid (RNA).

▶▶ Enhances the metabolism and synthesis of endogenous proteins.

▶▶ Facilitates the conversion of vitamins B2 and B3 to active endogenous coenzyme form.

Magnesium

Magnesium is the fourth most abundant mineral in the body. The magnesium ion is essential to all living cells and for good health. Approximately 50% of total body magnesium is found in bone. The other half is found predominantly inside cells of body tissues and organs. Only 1% of magnesium is found in blood, but the body works very hard to keep blood levels of magnesium constant. The adult human body contains about 25 grams of magnesium. Magnesium is needed for more than 300 biochemical reactions in the body. It helps maintain normal muscle and nerve function, keeps heart rhythm steady, supports a healthy immune system, and keeps bones strong.

Magnesium also helps regulate blood sugar levels, promotes normal blood pressure, and is known to be involved in energy metabolism and protein synthesis. It is required at a number of steps during the synthesis of nucleic acids (DNA and RNA) and proteins. A number of enzymes participating in the synthesis of carbohydrates and lipids require magnesium for their activity. Glutathione, an important antioxidant, requires magnesium for its synthesis as well. Magnesium is essential for muscle relaxation, protein synthesis, energy production on a cellular level, and nerve excitability. It is excreted through the kidneys.

Magnesium is absorbed into the body primarily from the ileum of the entire length of the small intestines. It is also absorbed via the colon. Magnesium requires an acidic stomach environment for absorption; supplements should therefore be consumed at bedtime or otherwise between meals — not at the same time as meals when the stomach's environment is alkaline. Hydrochloric acid is required for the absorption of the magnesium oxide form of magnesium. It is found in whole grain cereals, tofu, nuts, meat, milk, green vegetables, legumes, and chocolate.

*In normal muscle contraction calcium acts as a stimulator,
and magnesium as a relaxer.*

The proper balance of calcium, sodium, potassium, and magnesium maintains muscle tone and controls nerve irritability. The biological half-life for most magnesium that enters the body is between 41 and 181 days. There is a circadian rhythm associated with both the urinary excretion of magnesium and serum levels of magnesium. Maximum magnesium excretion occurs at night, while serum magnesium levels peak around midday. Magnesium is a carrier vehicle for the transport of calcium into and out of cell membranes (i.e. it facilitates the maintenance of calcium homeostasis). Magnesium prevents the accumulation of excessive quantities of calcium in the kidneys, a condition known as nephrocalcinosis. Magnesium enhances the function of phosphorus and is a carrier vehicle for the transport of potassium and sodium into and out of cell membranes.

Signs of deficiency include anorexia, growth failure, cardiac changes, neuromuscular changes, muscle weakness, irritability, and mental derangement. Osteoporosis can occur as a result of magnesium deficiency. Women afflicted with osteoporosis have been shown to have significantly lower bone magnesium than healthy women. Cirrhosis can also occur as a result of magnesium deficiency. Deficient levels of intracellular magnesium may contribute to the impaired insulin response that occurs in diabetes mellitus type 2 patients.

Signs of an overdose include diarrhea, transient hypocalcemia, respiratory paralysis, cardiac arrest, fatigue, depression, and decreased mental alertness.

Health benefits of magnesium

- ►► Improves the function of the adrenal glands.
- ►► Involved in the health of bones (64% of the body's magnesium is concentrated in the bones).
- ►► Modulates the electrical potential of cell membranes and maintains the permeability of cell membranes.
- ►► Helps to maintain the proper electrical charge gradient across cell membranes.
- ►► When combined with calcium, eliminates some types of toxic radioactive isotopes (radioisotopes) that may become lodged within the bones.
- ►► Alleviates heartburn.
- ►► In the magnesium aspartate form, lowers total serum cholesterol levels.
- ►► Raises HDL cholesterol levels and lowers serum LDL cholesterol levels.
- ►► Helps to prevent diabetes mellitus and to keep diabetes mellitus under control.

Sodium, chloride, and potassium

Electrolytes are substances that become ions in solution and acquire the capacity to conduct electricity. The balance of the electrolytes in our bodies is essential for normal function of our cells and our organs.

Sodium, chloride, and potassium are absorbed in the intestine. Sources include table salt, seafood, milk, and eggs. Potassium is found in fruit.

Signs of deficiency are not common but could include hypokalemia, lethargy, and muscle weakness.

A sign of overdose would include high blood pressure.

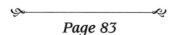

Sulfur

Sulfur is a non-metallic acidic macro mineral usually consumed as part of larger compounds rather than as elemental sulfur. Sulfur is the third most abundant mineral, based on percentage of total body weight. It can be found as a pure element or as sulfide and sulfate minerals. It is an essential element for life and is found in two amino acids, cysteine and methionine.

It is needed for synthesis of essential metabolites and functions in oxidation/reduction reactions.

Sources include protein foods such as meat, fish, poultry, eggs, milk, cheese, legumes, and nuts.

Signs of deficiency are not common; however, approximately 50% of the body's sulfur content is located in muscles. Osteoarthritis patients are often found to be deficient in sulfur (as measured by the cystine content of fingernails).

Health benefits of sulfur

- ▶▶ Facilitates the secretion of bile.
- ▶▶ Enhances the function and health of the pancreas.
- ▶▶ Is an essential component of antibodies.
- ▶▶ Kills or inhibits some forms of detrimental bacteria.
- ▶▶ Involved in the integrity of cartilage (the sulfur concentration in damaged cartilage is only 33% of the level of normal cartilage).
- ▶▶ Improves the function of the joints.
- ▶▶ Supplemental sulfur (either orally or via sulfur baths) alleviates the pain associated with osteoarthritis and restores endogenous sulfur levels to normal.
- ▶▶ Alleviates the pain and effusions that occur in rheumatoid arthritis.

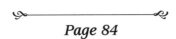

More Nutrients

Flavonoids

Bioflavonoids are a group of over 4,000 types of (usually) water-soluble compounds found in all vascular plants. All bioflavonoids are based on 15 carbon atoms that include a chromane ring bearing a second aromatic ring on the second, third, or fourth carbon. Bioflavonoids generally occur in dietary and herbal sources bound to carbohydrates (glucose, galactose, glucorhamnose, rhamnose, arabinose) as glycosides — collectively known as flavonglycosides.

During intestinal absorption, the free bioflavonoid is split off and released from the carbohydrate. Edema can occur as a result of bioflavonoid deficiency.

Most bioflavonoids increase the strength and resiliency of collagen. They protect and enhance the action of vitamin C and increase the absorption and bioavailability of orally administered vitamin C.

Polyphenol P

Polyphenols are found in all flowering plants. Many potently inhibit various forms of cancer because polyphenols prevent the conversion of nitrates and nitrites into carcinogenic nitrosamines within the stomach.

Indoles U

Indoles are a group of plant auxins (plant growth hormones) and can help to prevent some forms of cancer. Indoles help to prevent breast cancer by activating protective enzymes that deactivate the estrogens that are implicated in breast cancer. By retarding the ability of ingested or inhaled polynuclear aromatic hydrocarbons

(PAHs), indole keeps these substances from converting to cancer-causing substances within the liver.

Many dietary indoles possess antioxidant properties.

Peptides

Peptides are compounds consisting of two to 50 amino acids linked together.

Oligosaccharides

Oligosaccharides are a group of carbohydrates consisting of three to 15 monosaccharide molecules linked together and are a component of many endogenous glycoproteins and hormones. Endogenous oligosaccharides are produced during the digestion of many types of polysaccharides. Propionibacterium freudenreicvhii produces a bifidogenic growth stimulator (BGS) named ACNQ, which selectively enhances the utilization of oligosaccharides by bifidobacteria. Oligosaccharides are a constituent of many types of seeds.

Saponins

Saponins are a chemically diverse group of steroid-like glucoside glycoside terpenes. Most saponins lower total serum cholesterol by facilitating the binding of polysaccharides to bile acids.

Hippuric acid

Hippuric acid is a type of organic acid that helps to prevent and control urinary tract infections (UTIs), such as (bacterial) cystitis, by inhibiting the detrimental bacteria, especially eschericia coli, which cause UTIs.

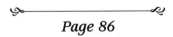

Hippuric acid is manufactured endogenously via the metabolism of benzoic acid and quinic acid. For example, the benzoic acid and quinic acid contained in cranberries metabolizes to hippuric acid when cranberries are ingested. Although the cranberry does not contain hippuric acid, the benzoic acid and quinic acid content of the cranberry metabolizes within the body to form hippuric acid.

Isoflavones

Isoflavonoids are a class of bioflavonoids. Isoflavonoids are also classified as phytoestrogens due to their ability to bind to estrogen receptors, which prevents true estrogens from occupying these receptors. Isoflavonoids, by binding to estrogen receptors and preventing the binding of true estrogens to these receptors, counteract estrogen hormones' cancer causing potential. Isoflavonoids are particularly effective for the prevention of breast cancer and possess antioxidant properties.

Forty mg per day of isoflavonoids derived from soybeans increases HDL cholesterol, lowers total serum cholesterol levels, and lowers LDL cholesterol levels. Isoflavonoids also help to prevent osteoporosis.

Carotenoids

Carotenoids are a family of more than 700 naturally occurring yellow, red, and orange pigments found in vegetables and fruits. (Specific carotenoids have also been identified in bird feathers and crustaceans.) Carotenoids are always present in photosynthetic plant tissues, being accessory pigments for chlorophyll. High quantities are also found in other plant tissues. Carotenoids absorb light in the 400-500 nm region of the visible light spectrum of the ultra-violet spectrum. This physical property is responsible for the characteristic pigmentation of the carotenoids.

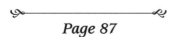

Glucosinolates

Glucosinolates are a group of pungent sulfuric compounds that are found almost exclusively in various plants from the cabbage (cruciferae) family. Approximately 100 different types of glucosinolates are known to exist in the plant kingdom, but only 10 are present in the cabbage family of vegetables. Glucosinolates kill the detrimental aflatoxin and block the development of (i.e. help to prevent) some forms of cancer.

Glucosinolates possess antioxidant properties. When the plant tissues of foods containing glucosinolates are disrupted (by chewing or cooking), the thioglucosidase enzyme (found in the tissues of glucosinolate containing plants) hydrolyzes glucosinolates to form the various categories of breakdown products of glucosinolates.

Sterols

Sterols are a group of steroid alcohol lipids in which the alcohol hydroxyl group is attached in position 3 and has an aliphatic side chain of at least eight carbon atoms at position 17. Most sterols have 29 carbon atoms. Types of sterols include cholesterol, phytosterols, and vitamin D.

Quinones

Quinones are a diverse group of compounds that have the structure of cyclic hydrocarbons with one or more benzene ring structures. Coenzymes Q are a class of fat-soluble quinones.

Types include anthraquinones, coenzymes Q, hydroquinones, idebenone, lapachol, pyrroloquinoline, quinone and vitamin K.

Biochanin A

Biochanin A is a type of isoflavonoid. It possesses antioxidant

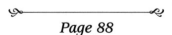

properties and is metabolized within the body to form genistein. Biochanin A counteracts potentially toxic substances and inhibits the activity of 5-alpha reductase in genital tissue. It can be found in beer and red clover.

Phospholipids (phosphatides)

Phospholipids are waxy, oily, endogenous, or exogenous compounds that are midway between lipids and water in density. Phospholipids are a component of every cell of the body but comprise less than 5% of the total lipids within the body. Endogenous phospholipids are manufactured in the liver. Phospholipids comprise 45% of the cell membranes of red blood cells and tissues within the body. They are especially prevalent in the brain. Phospholipids comprise 80% of the myelin sheaths that function as cell membranes for neurons in the brain. Phospholipids surround the mitochondria, nucleus, nucleolus, and lysosomes and form the membranous structures of golgi and endoplasmic reticulum.

The phospholipid component of cell membranes keeps water-insoluble fatty acids, cholesterol, vitamin A, and vitamin E soluble in the watery bloodstream. Phospholipids help to determine which substances can drift (or be pulled into) cells from outside and which substances from within cells will drift or be pushed out; therefore, they are involved in the regulation of the body's water balance. Phospholipids hold endogenous proteins in place in cell membranes to fulfill their structural, enzymatic, and transport functions. They form a barrier that keeps toxins outside of each cell.

Consumption of dietary phospholipids can strengthen cell membranes and make it harder for viruses to "steal" the membrane that they need to survive. Phospholipids are a nourishing agent for skin, particularly tired, dull skin.

Phospholipids are transported around the body by lipoproteins and are comprised of 7% of chylomicrons, 18% of very low

The EPA considers cadmium to be a probable human carcinogen (cancer-causing agent) and has classified it as a Group B1 carcinogen. The EPA uses mathematical models, based on animal studies, to estimate the probability of a person developing cancer from breathing air containing a specified concentration of a chemical. The agency calculated an inhalation unit risk estimate of $1.8 \times 10\text{-}3(\mu g/m3)$ and estimates that, if an individual were to continuously breathe air containing cadmium at an average of 0.0006 µg/m3 (6 x 10-7 mg/m3) over his or her entire lifetime, that person would theoretically have no more than a one-in-a-million increased chance of developing cancer as a direct result of breathing air containing this chemical.

Similarly, the EPA estimates that continuously breathing air containing 0.006 µg/m3 (6 x 10-6 mg/m3) would result in not greater than a one-in-a-hundred-thousand increased chance of developing cancer. Air containing 0.06 µg/m3 (6 x 10-5 mg/m3) would result in not greater than a one-in-ten-thousand increased chance of developing cancer.

• •

For a detailed discussion of confidence in the potency estimates, please see IRIS. Since we live in a polluted world, items like the battery in your car or fertilizers (es super-phosphates) can contain 15 to 21 milligrams of cadmium per kilogram. The lining of cans, dental material, some pharmaceuticals, confectioneries, cola, margarine, tobacco, and tap water.

density lipoprotein, 22% of low density lipoprotein (LDL), 22% of high density lipoprotein (HDL), and 22% of lipoprotein.

Phospholipases facilitate the digestion of dietary phospholipids. Vitamin A protects the fatty acids contained in phospholipids from oxidation damage.

Regular consumption of oily fish increases the super unsaturated fatty acid (especially the docosahexaenoic acid [DHA] and eicosapentaenoic acid [EPA]) content of serum phospholipids.

Simple sugars

Also known as simple carbohydrates (which always should be avoided), simple sugars are a group of monosaccharides and disaccharides.

Glucose is a carbohydrate and is the most important simple sugar in human metabolism. Glucose is called a simple sugar or a monosaccharide because it is one of the smallest units that has the characteristics of this class of carbohydrates. Glucose is sometimes called dextrose. Corn syrup is primarily glucose. Glucose is one of the primary molecules which serve as energy sources for plants and animals. It is found in the sap of plants and is found in the human bloodstream, where it is referred to as "blood sugar."

The normal concentration of glucose in the blood is about 0.1%, but it becomes much higher in persons suffering from diabetes.

Glucose entering the digestive tract lacks nutrients and it cannot be used by the body. High levels of glucose are also very toxic to the pancreas. The pancreas reacts by overproducing insulin to get rid of the glucose as fast as possible. Insulin over-production inhibits the function of glycogen synthase, which then cannot direct all glucose to healthy cells. Glucose, instead, will be directed to fat cells and eventually insulin resistance will occur and consequently diabetes is the final outcome.

Consuming foods poor in essential nutrients will not satisfy nutritional requirements for the body. Being nutritionally unsatisfied, we feel that hunger as a sugar craving sooner than the normal 3 to 3½ hours that should exist between meals. This leads to sugar addiction or sugar craving, similar to carbohydrate addiction syndrome. Excess sugar in the body is turned to fat by the liver.

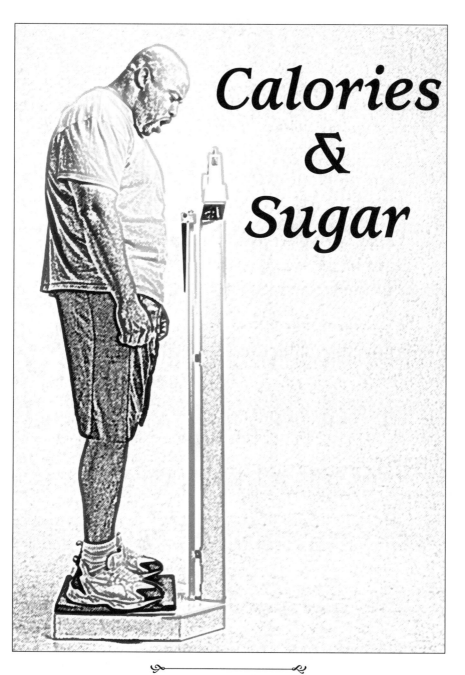

Calories
&
Sugar

Calories

One pound of body fat correlates to 3500 Kcal calories, a measurement of energy. In other words, to lose a pound of fat, one has to spend or burn 3500 calories more than what one consumes. Calories come in three flavors:

▸▸Carbohydrates or sugars
▸▸Proteins made of amino acids
▸▸Fats

1 gram of sugar provides 4 Kcal of energy.
1 gram of protein provides 9 Kcal of energy.
1 gram of fat provides 9 Kcal of energy.

Protein is less efficiently digested and absorbed, and a handling cost related to the energy the body has to spend to absorb the protein results in one gram of protein providing 20% less energy to the body than sugar. This is why most weight loss programs recommend reducing fat in the diet and replacing it with protein, such as tuna in water or chicken breast.

If you under-eat by 350 Kcal per day, you will lose a pound of fat every 10 days, or three pounds a month. The inverse is true as well. On the average, over-eating by 350 Kcal per day will cause a weight gain of about three pounds a month.

Toxic effects

Simple sugars increase the body's production of adrenaline by up to 400%. Excessive consumption of simple sugars accelerates the aging process by causing cross-linking (glycosylation) of the body's proteins.

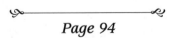

Excessive consumption also increases the risk of atherosclerosis because simple sugars cause cross-linking of the collagen that is a constituent of blood vessels.

Excessive consumption of simple sugars exacerbates irritable bowel syndrome by reducing the buffering effect of polysaccharides. Too much also damages the kidneys because simple sugars cause cross-linking of the collagen that is a component of the tiny filters within the kidneys. Excessive consumption increases the risk of cataracts and can accelerate the development of food allergies.

Simple sugars feed cancer cells and detrimental candida albicans yeast.

The immune system will try to suppress with excessive consumption of simple sugars, and simple sugars impair the ability of neutrophils to function as phagocytes.

Too much simple sugar causes the production of excessive quantities of acetic acid, which further contributes to excessive production of endogenous cholesterol. It can lower HDL cholesterol production. Simple sugars cause the cross-linking of the body's endogenous proteins — cross-linking with the body's proteins is known as glycosylation.

Excessive simple sugars are converted to triglycerides and are then stored within the body as adipose tissue (fat). This in turn causes fatigue and stimulates the production of free radicals. Too much also causes the body's joints to become brittle and stiffer because simple sugars cause cross-linking of the collagen that is a component of the joints.

Simple sugars can interact with detrimental bacteria that reside on the teeth (streptococcus mutants and streptococcus sobrinus) and result in the production of lactic acid, which causes tooth decay. Excessive consumption reduces the buffering effects of polysaccharides and contributes to linoleic acid deficiency by preventing its release from the body's adipose tissue.

Excessive consumption of simple sugars increases the body's excretion of magnesium and potassium. It causes the cross-linking of hemoglobin, thereby reducing the ability of hemoglobin to transport oxygen to red blood cells within the body.

Simple sugars cause the depletion of the body's vitamin B6 reserves and interfere with the transport of vitamin C through the body, as simple sugars use the same transport system as vitamin C. Soft drinks account for one-third of all dietary simple sugar consumption in the U.S.A. Hypoglycemia increases the craving for simple sugars.

Glucose

Monosaccharide sugar, also known as $C_6H_{12}O_6$, is found in honey and the juices of many fruits. The alternate name, grape sugar, is derived from the presence of glucose in grapes. It is the sugar most often produced by hydrolysis of natural glycosides. Glucose is a normal constituent of the blood of animals. It is a white crystalline solid, less sweet than ordinary table sugar. Solutions of glucose rotate the plane of polarization of polarized light to the right; hence the alternative name dextrose (Latin dexter, "right").

Glucose crystallizes in three different forms. The degree of rotation of polarized light is different for each form. Glucose is formed by the hydrolysis of many carbohydrates, including sucrose, maltose, cellulose, starch, and glycogen. Fermentation of glucose by yeast produces ethyl alcohol and carbon dioxide. Glucose is made industrially by the hydrolysis of starch under the influence of dilute acid or, more commonly, under that of enzymes. It is chiefly used as a sweetening agent in the food-processing industries. It is also used in tanning, in dye baths, in making tabulated products, and in medicine for treating dehydration and for intravenous feeding.

Sugars

The average American consumes an astounding two to three pounds of sugar each week, which is not surprising considering that highly refined sugars in the forms of sucrose (table sugar), dextrose (corn sugar), and high-fructose corn syrup are being processed into so many foods such as bread, breakfast cereal, mayonnaise, peanut butter, ketchup, spaghetti sauce, and a plethora of microwave meals.

In the last 20 years, we have increased sugar consumption in the U.S. from 26 pounds to 135 pounds of sugar per person per year! Prior to the turn of this century (1887-1890), the average consumption was only five pounds per person per year! Cardiovascular disease and cancer were virtually unknown in the early 1900's.

Sugar depresses the immune system and elevates insulin and triglyceride. We have known this for decades. It was only in the 1970's that researchers found out that vitamin C was needed by white blood cells so that they could phagocytes viruses and bacteria. White blood cells require a 50-times higher concentration inside the cell as outside, so they have to accumulate vitamin C.

There is something called a "phagocytic index," which tells you how rapidly a particular macrophage or lymphocyte can gobble up a virus, bacteria, or cancer cell. It was in the 1970's that Linus Pauling realized that white blood cells need a high dose of vitamin C, and that is when he came up with his theory that you need high doses of it to combat the common cold. Sugars interfere with the transport of vitamin C through the body.

One of sugar's major drawbacks is that it raises the insulin level, which inhibits the release of growth hormones, which in turn depresses the immune system. This is not something you want to take place if you want to avoid disease.

An influx of sugar into the bloodstream upsets the body's blood sugar balance, triggering the release of insulin, which the body uses to keep blood sugar at a constant and safe level. Insulin also promotes the storage of fat, so that when you eat sweets high in sugar, you're making way for rapid weight gain and elevated triglyceride levels, both of which have been linked to cardiovascular disease. Complex carbohydrates tend to be absorbed more slowly, lessening the impact on blood sugar levels.

Honey (a simple sugar)

There are four classes of simple sugars which are regarded by most naturopathic doctors and nutritionists as "harmful" substances: sucrose, fructose, honey, and malts.

Some of you may be surprised to find honey here. Although honey is a natural sweetener, it is considered a refined sugar because 96% of dry matter are simple sugars: fructose, glucose, and sucrose. Honey causes tooth decay faster than table sugar. Honey has the highest calorie content of all sugars with 65 calories/tablespoon, compared to the 48 calories/tablespoon found in table sugar.

Sucrose, beet sugar, cane sugar, table sugar, roots, and honey

Sucrose is a disaccharide comprising one molecule of fructose plus one molecule of glucose. Sucrase digests sucrose into its constituents — fructose and glucose — in the small intestine. It is the final product in photosynthesis and is used as a primary energy source in most organisms.

Sucrose interferes:

▸▸ Increases the body's excretion of calcium and chromium.
▸▸ Interferes with the absorption of magnesium and depletion of the body's phosphorus.
▸▸ Depletes the body's supply of biotin, choline, and vitamin B1.
▸▸ Interferes with the transport of vitamin C through the body.
▸▸ Increases the production of endogenous cholesterol, reduces HDL, and increases serum triglycerides.
▸▸ Increases the production of endogenous cortisol and uric acid.
▸▸ Digested very rapidly, which causes peaks and troughs in the body's blood sugar levels and causes the body to produce excessive amounts of insulin.

Toxic effects of sucrose
▸▸ Accelerates the aging process and accelerates the development of wrinkles (due to fructose and glucose in sucrose, stimulating the process of cross-linking).
▸▸ Increases blood pressure and therefore can contribute to the development of hypertension.
▸▸ Excessive consumption of sucrose has been related to Crohn's disease, and 80% of Crohn's disease patients who adopt a sucrose-free diet achieve an improvement in symptoms after 18 months.
▸▸ Excessive consumption of sucrose increases the risk of gallstones and kidney stones.
▸▸ Excessive consumption of sucrose interferes with the function of neutrophils and phagocytes by 50% acutely.
▸▸ Increases the risk of breast and colon cancers.
▸▸ Causes a temporary rise in blood sugar, which increases the body's production of insulin and can therefore contribute to insulin resistance.

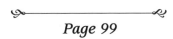

Fructose (fruit sugar or levulose)

Fructose is a type of hexose monosaccharide simple sugar carbohydrate that is twice as sweet as sucrose. Fructose is a component of sucrose (a disaccharide) and is a hexose (6-carbon sugar) that is a component of the disaccharide sucrose, a major plant sugar.

Health benefits
(when fruits and vegetables are eaten fresh)

➤ Is the only substance presently known that can accelerate the clearance of alcohol (ethanol) from the bloodstream.
➤ Provides the necessary energy to give sperm its motility (as a component of the seminal plasma portion of semen).

Fructose is a component of:
A — Fructooligosaccharides (FOS)
B — Inulin (a polysaccharide)
C — Lactulose (a disaccharide)
D — Melezitose (a trisaccharide)

A ~ Fructooligosaccharides (FOS) are a group of (non-digestible) oligosaccharides composed of short chain polymers of fructose. They are composed of one molecule of sucrose and one to three molecules of fructose.

Dietary sources of FOS include beer, bananas, rye, oats, chicory (root), burdock, leeks, onions, tomatoes, garlic, asparagus, and Jerusalem artichoke.

B ~ Inulin is a fructose glycan polysaccharide comprised of linked units (polymers) of fructose. Dietary sources of inulin include

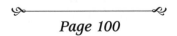

burdock, chicory, dandelion, echinacea, artichokes, and Jerusalem artichokes.

C ~ Lactulose is a type of disaccharide that consists of one molecule of galactose and one molecule of fructose. Dietary sources of lactulose include milk that is heated or stored, as lactulose does not occur naturally but is formed by isomerization.

D ~ Melezitose is a type of trisaccharide oligosaccharide, composed of two glucose molecules and one fructose molecule. It is hydrolyzed within the body to form glucose plus turanose (a disaccharide).

Toxic effects of fructose

Fructose accelerates the cross-linking of the skin's collagen content and the body's endogenous proteins more rapidly than glucose. It increases the risk of abnormal blood clotting ailments and is known to increase the risk of cardiovascular diseases. Fructose has been linked to calcium oxalate kidney stones, by increasing the concentration of calcium in the urine and increasing the urinary output of the N-acetyl-glucosaminidase enzyme that is only present in persons with kidney ailments.

Fructose interferes with the function of neutrophils and it serves in part as the raw material for the synthesis of cholesterol within the body. It actually increases total serum cholesterol, LDL cholesterol levels, and triglyceride levels.

Albumin is glycosylated 10 times as rapidly, and hemoglobin is glycosylated five times more rapidly with fructose than glucose. Fructose can cause insulin resistance with excessive consumption

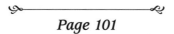

and it may increases the risk of gout since fructose increases the body's production of uric acid.

High fructose corn syrup (HFCS)

From 1970 to 1977, the annual per capita consumption of high fructose corn syrup (HFCS) in the United States increased from 0.5 pounds to 62.4 pounds. Sucrose consumption decreased from 102 pounds to 67 pounds per year.

Fructose is a type of hexose monosaccharide simple sugar carbohydrate and is twice as sweet as sucrose. If you see HFCS on a food label be aware that:

▶ HFCS is very sweet and increases fat production in the body.

▶ HFCS is based on the chemical compound of fructose and is very addictive.

▶ HFCS contains 97 % monosaccharides (55 % fructose, 42 % glucose), which is absorbed more rapidly and is a reducing sugar.

Types of sugar

▶ Sucrose is a disaccharide of glucose and fructose and not a reducing sugar. It requires hydrolysis by the gut disaccharides to be absorbed.

▶ Monosaccharides are a group of simple sugars that contain between three and nine carbon atoms — simple sugars are also known as simple carbohydrates.

▶ Disaccharides are a group of simple sugars that are a combination of two monosaccharides.

Sugar is bad enough, but it can be even more toxic when it is caramelized (cooked at a high temperature).

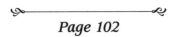

This transformation of sugar is referred to as the browning reaction, also called the Maillard reaction (AGE).

The Maillard reaction is a non-enzymatic browning reaction, caused by the condensation of an amino group and a reducing compound, resulting in complex changes in biological and food systems. This reaction was described for the first time by Louis Maillard in 1912. Maillard reaction occurs when virtually all foods are heated, and also occurs during storage. Most of the effects of the Maillard reaction, including the caramel aromas and golden brown colors, are desirable. Nevertheless, some of the effects of the Maillard reaction, including food darkness and off-flavor development, are undesirable.

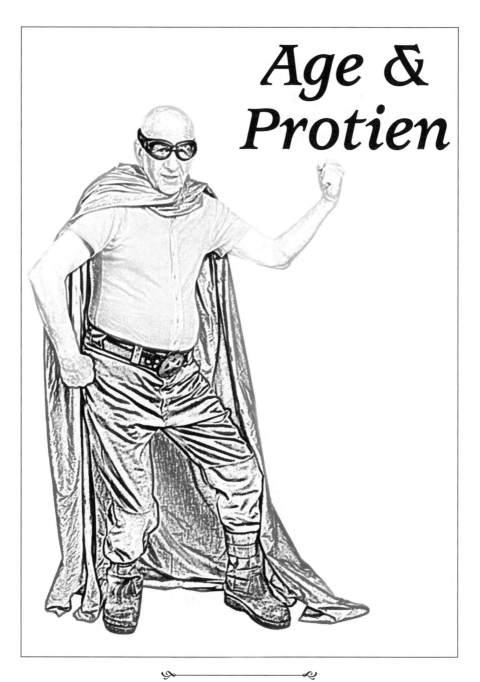

Age & Protien

AGE

Reducing sugar, plus amino acid, plus heat creates advanced glycation end product (or AGE) as a result of a chain of chemical reactions. AGE accumulates in many tissues during aging and at an accelerated rate during the course of diabetes. AGE causes cross-linking of long-lived proteins and contributes to the age-related decline in the function of cells and tissues that occurs in normal aging.

Accelerating the aging process

Cross-linking is an oxidation reaction in which bonds form between endogenous carbohydrates, nucleic acids, proteins, and lipids. The bonds formed during cross-linking can be between the same or different carbohydrates, proteins, nucleic acids, or lipids. This oxidation reaction is involved in the pathogenesis of atherosclerosis and is a complication of diabetes. Excessive cross-linking in the kidneys is responsible for diabetic neuropathy (blindness). C-reactive protein increases by 35% on a high-AGE diet and decreases by 20% on a low-AGE diet.

There are several substances that can reverse or prevent cross-linking. These substances include:
- Acetyl-L-Carnitine (ALC)
- Arginine
- Lysine
- Taurine
- Chromium (chromium picolinat)
- Inositol, lipoic acid, nicotinic acid, para aminobenzoic acid
- Vitamin A
- Vitamin B1, B5, B6

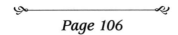

▸▸ Vitamin C
▸▸ Vitamin E

C-reactive protein (CRP)

C-reactive protein is a type of endogenous protein that is an acute phase reactant. It is produced in the liver and released in response to acute injury, bacterial and viral infection, or other stimulants of inflammation. C-reactive protein is synthesized exclusively in the liver and is secreted in increased amounts within six hours of an acute inflammatory stimulus. The plasma level can double at least every eight hours, reaching a peak after about 50 hours. After effective treatment or removal of the inflammatory stimulus, levels can fall almost as rapidly as the five- to seven-hour plasma half-life of labeled exogenous CRP. The only condition that interferes with the "normal" CRP response is severe hepatocellular impairment.

C-reactive protein is a biomarker (a sign) for:

1- Atherosclerosis
2- Blood clotting
3- Inflammation occurring in the lining of the arteries
4- Dilated cardiomyopathy
5- Future heart attack (people with a high level of C-reactive protein are three times more likely to die from a future heart attack)
6- Intermittent claudication
7- Future stroke (people with high level of C-reactive protein are seven times more likely to die from a future stroke)
8- Crohn's disease
9- Pancreatitis
10- Weakened immune system

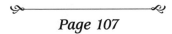

11- Bacterial and viral infections

12- Lymphoma

13- Rheumatic fever

14- Sarcomas

15- Insulin resistance

16- Rheumatoid arthritis

17- Fractures

Substances that lower C-reactive protein levels:

1- DHEA (Dehydroepiandrosterone)

2- Aspirin

3- Ibuprofen

4- Moderate consumption of alcohol

5- Vitamin B6

6- Vitamin C

7- Vitamin E toxins in our environment

Avoiding Toxins

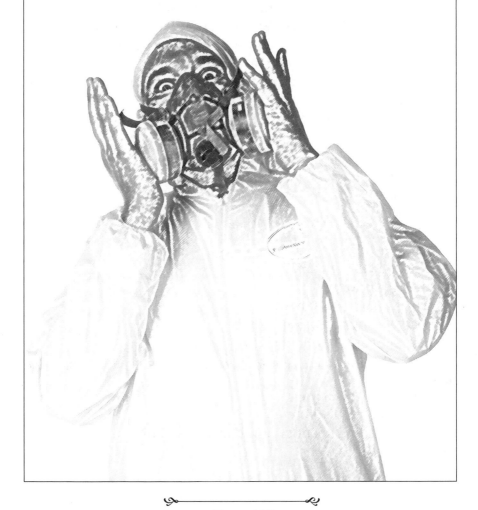

Avoiding Toxins

Pesticides

» Heptachlor induces several forms of cancer, including leukemia.
» Chlordane is a type of chlorinated hydrocarbon used as a pesticide, especially against termites. Chlordane has been banned for all purposes except for underground use against termites. It has been well proven to cause some forms of cancer, especially leukemia.
» Dioxin is a highly toxic constituent of the herbicide 2,4,5-T.

Others to avoid include:
1- Aspartame
2- Methanol
3- Formaldehyde
4- Cadmium
5- Arsenic
6- Lead
7- Mercury
8- Polyvinyl chloride (PVC)
9- Homogenization
10- Monosodium glutamate
11- Food additive/coloring agents
12- Sodium Lauryl Sulfate (SLS)
   Tartrazine, also known as Acid Yellow 23, C.I., 19140, FD&C Yellow No. 5, Filter
   Yellow, Food. Yellow No.4
12- Sodium metabisulfite
13- Potassium nitrite, potassium nitrate, sodium nitrite
14- Nitrosamines

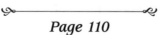

Enzymes are the key to life. No enzymes, no life. We destroy all the digestive enzymes in our food by cooking and baking, and thus the body has to draw the necessary enzymes to digest this dead food from the body organs, which in turn become unbalanced, leaving the majority of people in this country lacking enzymes. Digestive enzymes are made in the body (primarily in the pancreas). There are approximately 22 different digestive enzymes, and these continue the body's digestive process in the upper part of the small intestine. Eating enzyme-deficient foods can result in poor digestion and enzyme deficiencies.

The signs of enzyme deficiency are inflammation (pain and swelling), fatigue, headaches, sinus problems, allergies, colon problems, and arthritis/joint pain. In young adults, acne or ADD/ADHD can be an enzyme deficiency. Whatever food particles you do not digest will become toxins in your body.

Enzymes' specific jobs:
Digest food • Break down toxins
Cleanse the blood
Strengthen the immune system
Build protein into muscle
Contract muscles
Eliminate carbon dioxide from lungs
Reduce stress on the pancreas

Aspartame™

Aspartame contains alcohols, methanol, amino acids, aspartic acid, and phenylalanine. The FDA approved aspartame as a low-nutritive sweetener for use in solid form in 1981, and for use in soft drinks in 1983. It is a synthetic chemical consisting of two amino acids, phenylalanine (50%), aspartic acid (40%), and a methyl ester (10%) that promptly becomes free methyl alcohol (methanol, wood alcohol). The latter is universally considered a severe poison.

Links between aspartame and brain tumors were dismissed by the FDA cancer group. On November 18, 1996, the news organization CNN posted this on their Web site — "Several consumer groups Monday renewed their criticism of aspartame, citing a new study suggesting a possible link between the artificial sweetener and brain tumors.

But the Food and Drug Administration said both it and the National Cancer Institute have found 'no association between aspartame consumption and human brain tumors.'

Senior FDA scientists and consultants vigorously protested approving the release of aspartame products. Their objections related to disturbing findings in animal studies (especially the frequency of brain tumors), seemingly flawed experimental data, and the absence of extensive pre-marketing trials on humans using real-world products over prolonged periods."

Now you can ask what the job of FDA is; I hope it would be to protect us. Aspartame reactions may be caused by the compound itself. Reactions often occur in conjunction with severe caloric restriction and excessive exercise to lose weight. I suggest that you avoid aspartame at all costs. Eat sugar if you must, but not aspartame.

The compounds in aspartame can suppress the immune system, which can lead to diseases like lupus, multiple sclerosis, and fibromyalgia. Aspartame is marketed as NutraSweet, Equal, and Spoonful. In a keynote address by the EPA, it was announced that there was an epidemic of multiple sclerosis and systemic lupus. The EPA stated that they did not understand what toxin was causing this rampant epidemic across the United States. With over 5,000 products containing this chemical, perhaps it is no mystery.

When the temperature of aspartame exceeds 86°F, the wood alcohol in aspartame converts to formaldehyde and then to formic acid, which in turn causes metabolic acidosis. Formic acid is the poison found in the sting of fire ants. Multiple sclerosis is a disease of methanol toxicity and methanol toxicity mimics multiple sclerosis.

Fibromyalgia symptoms include: spasms, shooting pains, numbness in your legs, cramps, vertigo, dizziness, headaches, tinnitus, joint pain, depression, anxiety attacks, slurred speech, blurred vision, or memory loss. I would suggest you probably have ASPARTAME DISEASE!

The methanol in aspartame converts to formaldehyde in the retina of the eye. Formaldehyde is grouped in the same class of drugs as cyanide and arsenic — DEADLY POISONS!!!

Formaldehyde stores in the fat cells, particularly in the hips and thighs.

Aspartame is especially deadly for diabetics. All physicians know what wood alcohol will do to a diabetic. We find that physicians believe that they have patients with retinopathy, when in fact, it is caused by the aspartame. The aspartame keeps the blood sugar level out of control, causing many patients to go into a coma.

Often diabetics use aspartame to replace sugar. This fake sugar can actually cause diabetes to be irreversible in early stages of the disease. It is inexcusable that aspartame has been advertised as a substitute for sugar when it is so damaging.

Aspartic acid and phenylalanine are the by products your body produces from ingesting aspartame. Both are neurotoxic without the other amino acids found in protein because they mimic what a true amino acid should be. Aspartic acid and phenylalanine can cause memory loss and brain damage of varying degrees. Additionally, phenylalanine in aspartame breaks down the seizure threshold and depletes serotonin, which causes manic depression, panic attacks, rage, and violence.

Aspartame can cause:
1- Multiple sclerosis
2- Brain cancer

3- Systemic lupus erythematous (SLE)

4- Diabetes mellitus (cataracts, diabetic neuropathy, diabetic retinopathy)

5- Grave's disease

6- Headaches

7- Depression

8- Anxiety

9- Convulsions

10- Hearing loss

11- Joint pain

12- Fatigue

13- Insomnia

14- Memory impairment

15- Irritability

16- Migraine

18- Nausea

19- Symptoms resembling multiple sclerosis (due to the methanol content of aspartame)

20- Neuralgia (due to methanol)

21- Neuritis (due to methanol)

22- Neuropathy (due to methanol)

23- Damage the optic nerve and eventually blindness (due to methanol)

24- Numbness

25- Loss of sense of taste

26- Tinnitus

27- Vertigo

28- Asthma

28- Male impotence (There are reports of cases of male impotence that have resolved completely following the withdrawal of aspartame use.)

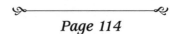

Alternatives

Stevia is a small perennial shrub that belongs to the chrysanthemum family of plants and is native to Paraguay. Stevia has the natural ability to sweeten and is approximately 15 times sweeter than common table sugar.

Stevia may well be the most remarkable sweetener in the world, but should not be overused.

The unique properties of Stevia were first identified in 1908, and by 1931 Stevia was being crystallized for use in foods, beverages, and pharmaceuticals.

Stevia has been used by native Indians since pre-Columbian times as an additive to their medicines and teas. Stevia currently makes up approximately 40% of Japan's sweetener market and consumption today. Stevia is the perfect alternative for those wishing to watch their caloric intake and who are concerned about the reported health risks of aspartame (NutraSweet) and saccharin (Sweet'N Low).

The following are some of the characteristics of Stevia:

- ▸▸ Safe for diabetics
- ▸▸ Calorie free
- ▸▸ Does not adversely affect blood sugar
- ▸▸ Non-toxic
- ▸▸ Inhibits the formation of cavities and plaque
- ▸▸ Contains no artificial ingredients
- ▸▸ Easy to use for cooking

Methanol

Methanol is a colorless, extremely toxic primary alcohol and is also known as carbinol, Columbian spirits, methyl alcohol, methylol, wood alcohol, wood naptha, and wood spirit.

Methanol is a component of the artificial sweetener aspartame and is responsible for many of the toxic effects of aspartame consumption. Methanol causes tinnitus, damages the optic nerve, and can cause blindness.

Methanol can damage the thymus gland (due to its metabolism to formaldehyde and formic acid within the body).

Methanol causes headaches, nausea, neuralgia, neuritis, and neuropathy. Ingested methanol is metabolized by the liver to form formaldehyde and formic acid. It is absorbed efficiently and has a very low rate of excretion; therefore, it is regarded as a cumulative toxin.

Formaldehyde

Formaldehyde is a colorless, gaseous aldehyde. It is both naturally occurring and a human-made compound. It is a gas with a pungent, suffocating odor at room temperature. You can smell formaldehyde at 830 parts of formaldehyde per billion parts of air. Formaldehyde is naturally formed from burning wood in forest fires and wood stoves. It also occurs in cigarette smoke. Until 1982, when it was banned, urea-formaldehyde was used as an insulating material in many homes in the United States. Formaldehyde is mainly used in chemical manufacturing processes. It is also used in agriculture as an analytical reagent, in concrete and plaster additives, cosmetics, disinfectants, fumigants, photography, and wood preservation. Formaldehyde is a common glue in wood products such as plywood and particle board.

Toxic effects of formaldehyde
➤ Causes cancer in rats.
➤ Potentates the toxicity of radiation in human lungs.
➤ Damages the thymus gland.
➤ Is toxic to the central nervous system.
➤ Reduces concentration ability.
➤ Can cause depression.
➤ Causes problems with memory.

Cadmium

Cadmium is a type of toxic micro-mineral. It is a heavy metal. As a solid, cadmium is silver-white, blue-tinged, and lustrous. As a fume, cadmium is odorless, yellow-brown, and very fine. Cadmium is used as a pigment. It can also be released during many other operations, such as welding, cutting, burning, drilling, or sandblasting of stainless steel or surfaces containing old paint. Cadmium may be used as a blue-white malleable metal or as a grayish-white powder.

The main sources of cadmium in the air are the burning of fossil fuels such as coal or oil, and the incineration of municipal waste. The acute (short-term) effects of cadmium in humans through inhalation exposure consist mainly of effects on the lungs, such as pulmonary irritation. Chronic (long-term) inhalation or oral exposure to cadmium leads to a build-up of cadmium in the kidneys that can cause kidney disease. Cadmium has been shown to be a developmental toxicant in animals, resulting in fetal malformations and other effects. An association between cadmium exposure and an increased risk of lung cancer has been reported in human studies, but these studies are inconclusive due to confounding factors. Animal studies have demonstrated an increase in lung cancer from long-term inhalation exposure to cadmium. The EPA has classified cadmium as a Group B1, probable human carcinogen.

Cadmium causes bone loss in experimental animals at blood cadmium concentrations below current OSHA standards for industrial exposure (USOSHA92). The largest sources of airborne cadmium in the environment are the burning of fossil fuels such as coal or oil, and incineration of municipal waste materials. Cadmium may also be emitted into the air from zinc, lead, or copper smelters.

For non-smokers, food is generally the largest source of cadmium exposure. Cadmium levels in some foods can be increased by the application of phosphate fertilizers or sewage sludge to farm fields.

Smoking is another important source of cadmium exposure. Smokers have about twice as much cadmium in their bodies as non-smokers.

Persons who smoke one or more packs of cigarettes per day show mean blood cadmium concentrations (2 ug/l) tenfold over those of non-smokers (about 0.2 ug/l) — in range of blood concentrations causing bone loss in animals. Cadmium in cigarettes may be an important cause of osteoporosis in humans.

Chronic effects (non-cancer)

Chronic inhalation and oral exposure to cadmium in humans results in a build-up of cadmium in the kidneys that can cause kidney disease, including proteinuria (a decrease in kidney's filtration rate), and an increased frequency of kidney stone formation. Chronic inhalation or oral exposure to cadmium in animals results in effects on the kidney, liver, lung, bone, immune system, blood, and nervous system.

The reference dose (RD) for cadmium in drinking water is 0.0005 milligrams per kilogram per day (mg/kg/d) and the RD for dietary exposure to cadmium is 0.001 mg/kg/d; both are based on the measurement of protein in urine in humans. The RD is an estimate of daily oral exposure to the human population (including sensitive subgroups) that is not likely to be carcinogenic during a lifetime. It is not a direct estimator of risk, but rather a reference point to gauge the potential effects. At exposures increasingly greater than the RD, the potential for adverse health effects increases. Lifetime exposure above the RD does not imply that an adverse health effect would necessarily occur.

The California Environmental Protection Agency has established a chronic reference exposure level of 0.00001 milligrams per cubic meter (mg/m3) for cadmium based on kidney and respiratory effects in humans.

Cadmium is highly toxic; it is more toxic than lead or mercury.

Toxic effects of cadmium exposure:
- Lowers thyroid activity.
- Decreases the level of glutathione present in the liver.
- Causes cross-linking of the body's endogenous nucleic acids, proteins, and lipids.
- Stimulates the production of free radicals.
- Damages the liver.
- Interferes with bone formation.
- Can cause osteomalacia and osteoporosis.
- Can cause male infertility.
- Is strongly implicated as a cause of enlarged prostate.
- Raises blood pressure (via kidney damage).
- Increases the incidence of calcium kidney stones.
- Reduces the body's production of some types of antibodies.
- Increases susceptibility to bacterial and viral diseases.
- Increases the risk of prostate cancer (due to its antagonism of zinc and selenium cadmium, which can replace zinc in the prostate).

Cancer risk

Several occupational studies have reported an excess risk of lung cancer in humans from exposure to inhaled cadmium. However, the evidence is limited rather than conclusive due to confounding factors. Animal studies have reported cancer resulting from inhalation exposure to several forms of cadmium, while animal ingestion studies have not demonstrated cancer resulting from exposure to cadmium compounds.

Arsenic

Arsenic is a type of toxic mineral. The average daily arsenic intake in adults is 0.5-1.0mg. Arsenic is a widely distributed element and is found in many ores, soils, and mineral waters. Currently, arsenic is used primarily in the production of glass and semiconductors, in wood and hide preservation, and as an additive to metal alloys to increase hardening and heat resistance. In the past arsenic was used as weed killer, rodenticide, in chemical warfare, and in the production of pigments and enamels.

Arsenic compounds are now rarely used in medicine, although some organic compounds of arsenic are used in the treatment of trypanomiasis and amoebiasis. The inorganic forms of arsenic are more toxic than the organic forms, and the trivalent forms are more toxic than the pentavalent forms. Arsenic can be inhaled, absorbed through the skin, or absorbed in the GI tract after ingestion. After a very small dose of arsenic (like those experienced daily by most people), most of the absorbed inorganic arsenic undergoes methylation mainly in the liver, to monomethylarsonic acid and dimethylarsinic acid, which are excreted along with residual inorganic arsenic in the urine. However, if the dose of arsenic is very large, the elimination half-life is prolonged.

Once absorbed, arsenic rapidly combines with the globin portion of hemoglobin and therefore localizes in the blood. There is minimal penetration of the blood-brain barrier, and within 24 hours arsenic redistributes itself to the liver, kidney, spleen, lung, and GI tract, with lesser accumulation in muscle and nervous tissue.

The mechanism of toxicity of all arsenic-containing compounds is the same. Once in the tissues, arsenic exerts its toxic effect through several mechanisms, the most significant of which is that it keeps cells from producing energy.

The average human body contains a total of 10 to 20 mg of arsenic.
The average safe organic arsenic daily consumption is 1 mg per day.
The lethal dosage of arsenic is 100 mg (of arsenic trioxide).

The toxic effects of arsenic include
▸ Damages or kills cells by causing aberrations to chromosomes.
▸ Increases the risk of bladder cancer.
▸ Accumulates in the spleen and liver.

Arsenic poisoning causes fatigue, goiter, jaundice, numbness, vertigo, headaches, nausea, memory impairment, dermatitis, and eczema.

Food source

Dairy products can contribute as much as 31% of arsenic in the diet; meat, poultry, fish, grains, and cereal products collectively contribute approximately 56% (Mahaffey et al., 1975). Based on a national survey conducted in six Canadian cities from 1985 to 1988,

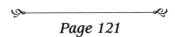

it was reported that foods containing the highest concentrations of arsenic were fish (1,662 ng/g), meat and poultry (24.3 ng/g), bakery goods and cereals (24.5 ng/g), and fats and oils (19 ng/g) (Dabeka et al., 1993). The substantial portion of arsenic present in fish is in the organic form. The major contributors of inorganic arsenic are raw rice (74 ng/g), flour (11 ng/g), grape juice (9 ng/g), and cooked spinach (6 ng/g) (Schoof et al., 1999).

Substances that help eliminate arsenic from the body
▸▸ Amino acids
▸▸ Minerals — zinc, calcium, magnesium, selenium, and iodine
▸▸ Vitamin C

Humans are exposed to mercury primarily in two forms, mercury vapor and methyl mercury compounds. Unfortunately mercury is a ubiquitous substance in our environment. Mercury vapor in the atmosphere makes its way into fresh and salt water by falling in precipitation. Methyl mercury compounds are created by bacterial conversion of inorganic mercury in water and soil, which subsequently concentrates in seafood and fish. Dietary fish intake has been found to have a direct correlation with methyl mercury levels in blood and hair of humans.

Silver amalgam dental fillings are the major source of inorganic mercury exposure in humans. This term, however, is a misnomer as this compound is not predominately silver. The proper term should be mercury amalgam. The most common dental filling material, amalgams contain approximately 50% liquid metallic mercury, 35% silver, 9% tin, 6% copper, and a trace of zinc. As this filling material is prepared and placed in the patient's mouth, the dentist and the person preparing the amalgam, along with the patient, are exposed to mercury vapor (HgO). The patient is further exposed to mercury vapor as the amalgam releases HgO when the individual chews, brushes, or drinks hot beverages.

Studies of mercury content in the exhaled air of those with and without amalgams have found significantly higher baseline mercury levels in subjects with amalgams and up to a 15.6-fold increase in mercury in exhaled air after chewing. Mercury release was found to be greater in corroded amalgams compared to new, polished fillings. Mercury vapor from amalgams enters the bloodstream after being inhaled into the lungs.

Comparisons of blood levels of mercury and the number of filings you have show a direct correlation with the amount of mercury in your blood and urine. In addition, a statistically significant correlation was found between the number of dental amalgam fillings and mercury content of the kidney cortex ($p < 0.0001$) and the occipital lobe cortex of the brain ($p < 0.0016$) in cadavers.

After removal of all amalgams, there is a transient increase in mercury concentration in the blood, plasma, and feces, followed by a decrease in blood levels below the pre-removal baseline.

Mercury vapor is lipid-soluble, freely passing through cell membranes and across the blood-brain barrier (BBB). Methyl mercury also easily crosses the BBB and the placenta. Inorganic and methyl mercury have a high affinity for sulfhydryl, reacting intracellularly with the sulfhydryl group on glutathione, cysteine, and histidine residues in proteins, and allowing transport out of the cell. In rats, it was found that mercury secretion into the bile was dependent on glutathione secretion into the bile, suggesting the biliary secretion of glutathione (GSH). In humans, 90% of mercury elimination is via the feces, with only 10% normally being excreted in the urine. An increase in hepatic GSH content helps to excrete excess mercury.

Polyvinyl chloride (PVC)

PVC is a rigid plastic that is soft and flexible if compounded with plasticizing materials. Health wise, PVC is regarded as an environmental toxin. Heat increases the release of PVC into food; therefore, foods that are to be microwaved should not be wrapped in PVC wrapping material.

PVC is strongly suspected of causing some forms of cancer:
▸▸ Brain cancer
▸▸ Liver cancer
▸▸ Lung cancer
▸▸ Lymphomas

At Tufts Medical School in Boston in 1987, two researchers, Soto and Sonnenschein, serendipitously discovered that plastic test tubes thought to be inert contained a chemical that stimulated breast cancer cells to grow and proliferate wildly. They were experimenting with malignant breast cancer cells that were sensitive to estrogen. When exposed to estrogen the cells would grow and multiply, and when isolated from estrogen, the cells would stop multiplying.

During the course of their experiments, they found that the test tube manufacturer changed the formulation of the plastic test tubes that they were using. The manufacturer had used p-nonylphenol, one of the family of synthetic chemicals called alkylphenols, to make these plastics more stable and less breakable. Manufacturers routinely add nonlyphenols to polystyrene and polyvinyl chloride (PVC). These new plastic test tubes caused their estrogen-sensitive breast cancer cells to proliferate, multiply, and grow. Thus, they concluded that p-nonylphenol acted like an estrogen.

Today PVC is the second most popular plastic in the world.

Homogenization — possible toxic effects

Xanthine oxidase (XO) is a type of endogenous oxidase enzyme that normally passes through the body without absorption, unless

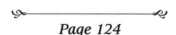

our digestion function is impaired. Some researchers propose that homogenization allows the absorption of XO (an enzyme naturally present in milk and cream) into the body. XO is a complex enzyme containing molybdenum, a bovine milk enzyme.

Researchers have purified human XO from breast milk and shown it to have properties that are surprisingly different from those of other mammalian XO. Elevated levels of circulating XO are characteristic of certain forms of liver and heart disease.

XO has a very specific function in our bodies. It breaks down purine compounds into uric acid, which is a waste product. The liver of several animals, including humans, contains XO specifically for this purpose.

Why homogenization?

Homogenization forces the milk, under extreme pressure, through tiny holes. This breaks up the normally large fat particles into tiny ones and forces the fat to form tiny molecular clusters, thus ensuring that the molecules do not regroup and form a cream layer on top of the milk. Instead, in this denatured state, they stay suspended in the milk. However, not only do they not regroup, the process also makes digestion almost impossible. The tiny molecules enter the bloodstream directly as undigested fat, not exactly the best for human health.

Toxic effects of xanthine oxidase include an increased risk of atherosclerosis. It has been speculated that dietary XO (when absorbed because of homogenization) contributes to the development of atherosclerosis. XO also facilitates the endogenous production of collagenase and elastase.

It stimulates the production of several types of free radicals including hydrogen peroxide and superoxide free radicals. XO stimulates lipid peroxidation within the skeletal muscles, an activity implicated in gout.

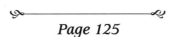

Monosodium glutamate (MSG)

Monosodium glutamate is the sodium (salt) of glutamic acid, an amino acid, which is a drug. It acts as an excitatory neurotransmitter and basically causes the nerve cells to discharge an electrical impulse that is the basis of its use as a flavor enhancer. Food companies learned that MSG could increase the flavor and aroma as well as enhance acceptability of commercial food products. Equally important, they learned that it could also suppress undesirable flavors, bitterness, and sourness is some foods. MSG can eliminate the "tinny" taste of canned foods. This is the reason food companies in general have no intention of giving up MSG as an additive in their products. U.S. national consumption of MSG went from roughly one million pounds in 1950 to 300 times that amount today. Here's the bottom line — as the dose increases, every single human will react to MSG at some point. At certain doses it becomes toxic enough to cause illness.

MSG is known to be more toxic than glutamic acid, as it is more readily absorbed by the body. There is some evidence that MSG in the doses most likely to be consumed by humans (i.e. 0.2% to 0.8% of processed foods) rarely causes the toxic effects listed below. Studies conducted on rats using 0.1% to 0.4% MSG caused no noticeable toxicity.

An excess consumption of MSG can cause intestinal cramps, nausea, vomiting, and convulsions, as well as blurred vision. MSG causes atrophy of the thyroid and pituitary gland. You can get an excess amount of MSG by consuming too much manufactured food over a long period of time. Be warned — some restaurants also use MSG. Just ask them.

Consumption of MSG can cause headaches
and trigger migraines.

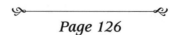

Many of the toxic effects of excessive consumption of MSG are due to MSG causing excessive stimulation of the N-methyl-D-aspartate receptors in the brain, causing vertigo. Consumption of MSG can also cause infertility in females and males, and atrophy of the ovaries and testes. MSG consumption has also been linked to fibermyalgia and depression.

Dioxin

Dioxin is a by-product of the manufacture, molding, or burning of organic chemicals and plastics that contain chlorine. It is the nastiest, most toxic man-made organic chemical. Its toxicity is second only to radioactive waste. The concern about dioxin is based on the fact that it persists in the environment and can accumulate in the body through the consumption of some foods containing fat. It occurs during the chlorine bleaching of wood pulp used to make paper, during the manufacture of chlorinated pesticides, and to a smaller extent it occurs naturally when forests and prairies burn.

Dioxin and dioxin-like chemicals such as PCBs and polyaromatic hydrocarbons, sometimes called xenoestrogens, happen when you microwave food in plastic or drink water in a soft plastic container that has been heated up.

These chemicals can be found in farm-raised fish. These chemicals can mimic estrogen, thereby disrupting the function of the sex hormone estrogen that your body would normally produce. They may also affect development of the immune system or cause cancer. Don't freeze your plastic water bottles with the water in them as this also releases dioxins in the plastic.

Dioxin has its toxic effect at the cellular level. In a complex pathway, dioxin interacts with DNA to alter how genes control protein synthesis.

It has also been linked to birth defects, immune system dysfunction, hormonal imbalances, male infertility, and other health problems. It rapidly builds up in the food chain and is known to contaminate human breast milk, cow's milk, and other dairy products, as well as fish in the Great Lakes. It is dangerous to those who consume these fish.

Toxic effects of dioxin are many. Dioxin competes with estrogens for attachment to the aryl hydrocarbon receptor located on certain cells. After dioxin has attached to this receptor, it is transported to the DNA of cells, where it binds to cellular proteins and causes the activation of genes that promote cancer. Therefore, dioxin exposure increases the risk of breast cancer and prostate cancer.

Dioxin is present in many processed foods including fried chicken, hamburgers, and ice cream.

Food coloring

Tartrazine is also known as Acid Yellow 23, C.I. 19140, FD&C Yellow No. 5, Filter Yellow, and Food Yellow No.4

Tartrazine is a coal-tar derivative that is used to color foods, cosmetics, and other products. It is literally industrial waste. It is most commonly used to provide the yellow or orange color of many processed foods.

Tartrazine is not just a color; it is a complex product containing many different chemical compounds. It is used in drugs, especially shells of medicinal capsules, syrups, cosmetics, fruit cordial, colored fizzy drinks, instant puddings, cake mixes, custard powder, soups, sauces, ice cream, popsicles, sweets, chewing gum, marzipan, jam, jelly, marmalade, mustard, yogurt, and many convenience foods together with glycerin, lemon, and honey products.

It can also be used with Brilliant Blue FCF to produce various green shades, especially for tinned processed peas.

Tartrazine has been implicated in some cases of attention deficit disorder (ADD), provoking symptoms in some children. In others, tartrazine induces asthma in those who are already susceptible. Tartrazine often causes hives.

Watch food labels for these chemical names:

4,5-dihydro-5-oxo-1-(4-sulfophenyl)-4-[(4-sulfophenyl)azo]-1H-Pyrazole-3-carboxylic acid, trisodium salt, Dihydro-5-oxo-1-(4-sulfophenyl)-4-[(4-sulfophenyl)azo]-1h-pyrazole-3-carboxylic acid, trisodium salt, Pyrazole-3-carboxylic acid, 4,5-dihydro-5-oxo-1-(4-sulfophenyl)-4-[(4-sulfophenyl)azo]-, trisodium salt, Sulfophenyl)-4-[(4-sulfophenyl)azo]-1h-pyrazole-3-carboxylic acid and trisodium salt, Trisodium 1-(4-sulfophenyl)-4-[(4-sulfophenyl)azo]-1h-pyrazole-3-carboxylate

Sodium metabisulfite (also known as sodium metabisulphite)

Sodium metabisulfite is used as a food additive, mainly as a preservative, and is sometimes identified as E223. As an additive, it may cause allergic reactions, particularly skin irritation, gastric irritation, and asthma. It is not recommended for consumption by children.

Sodium metabisulfite is used in a variety of processed foods during their manufacture — especially wine, beer, fruit juices, frozen apples, and dried fruits.

It causes severe allergies in some people and has caused anaphylactic shock that has resulted in death in rare cases. Sodium metabisulfite can induce asthma in susceptible individuals. It also causes the depletion of vitamin B1 in the body.

Potassium Nitrate
Sodium Nitrite

Adding nitrite to meat is only part of the curing process. Ordinary table salt (sodium chloride) is added because of its effect on flavor. Sugar is added to reduce the harshness of salt. Spices and other flavorings often are added to achieve a characteristic brand flavor. Most, but not all, cured meat products are smoked after the curing process to impart a smoked meat flavor. Sodium nitrite, rather than sodium nitrate, is most commonly used for curing (although in some products, such as country ham, sodium nitrate is used because of the long aging period). In a series of normal reactions, nitrite is converted to nitric oxide. Nitric oxide combines with myoglobin, the pigment responsible for the natural red color of uncured meat. Combined they form nitric oxide myoglobin, which is a deep red color (as in uncooked dry sausage) that changes to the characteristic bright pink normally associated with cured and smoked meat (such as wieners and ham) when heated during the smoking process.

Potassium nitrite is a type of nitrite that is commonly employed as a food preservative, while potassium nitrate is commonly employed as a synthetic food preservative and color fixative. It is also the active ingredient in most toothpaste designed for sensitive teeth.

Toxic effects of potassium and sodium nitrite and nitrate, when combined with amino acids within the stomach to form nitrosamines, are extremely potent carcinogens capable of causing cancer in many parts of the body.

Potassium nitrite can cause stomach cancer. Sodium nitrite can trigger migraines. Sodium nitrate interferes with the absorption of vitamin A.

Nitrosamines

Nitrosamines are a toxic group of amines. They are organic oxides of nitrogen that are formed within the body. Foods that contribute to the formation of nitrosamines are processed meats such as bacon, corned beef, frankfurters, ham, and salami.

Nitrosamines are extremely potent carcinogens which can cause cancer in any part of the body including the esophagus, larynx, lungs, mouth, and stomach.

Types of nitrosamines

- Methylnitrosamino-1-(3-pyridyl)-1-butanone (NNK) is present in tobacco smoke, is highly carcinogenic, and is implicated in lung cancer.
- N-nitrosodiethanolamine (NDELA) is present in many cosmetics and shampoos.
- N-nitrosodiethylamine and N-nitrosomorpholine are present in automobile interiors.
- N-nitrosodimethylamine (NDMA) is present in automobile interiors, beer, and scotch whiskey.
- N-nitrosohydroxypryyolidone is present in some processed meats.

Calcium carbide (artificial ripening)

An apple a day may keep the doctor away. However, those who consume local fruits on an almost daily basis may have to think twice before they bite into that ripe avocado or mango, as rather than keeping the doctor away, it's likely you would need to rush to your doctor. Until now a healthy diet has always been supplemented with the best of local fruits such as mango, plantain, papaw, pineapple, and avocado. These are so tempting when they are ripe.

What most of us do not know is that these fruits can severely affect our health. When you sometimes pay twice as much for a golden fruit and it still tastes watery, it could be possible that it has been treated with carbide. Don't fault the fruits for this. The blame lays with unscrupulous traders, who in a hurry to earn quick bucks, are resorting to a quick-fire but potentially poisonous method to ripen fruits in one to two days.

The fast ripening of fruits means they imbibe various harmful properties. The commonly used agent in the ripening process is calcium carbide, a material more commonly used for welding purposes.

The carbide is imported from countries such as China, Taiwan, and South Africa. Calcium carbide treatment is extremely hazardous because it contains traces of arsenic and phosphorous.

Once dissolved in water, the carbide produces acetylene gas. Acetylene gas is an analogue of the natural ripening agents produced by fruits known as ethylene. Acetylene imitates the ethylene and quickens the ripening process. In some cases it is only the skin that changes color, while the fruit itself remains green and raw. When the carbide is used on very raw fruit, the amount of the chemical needed to ripen the fruit has to be increased. This results in the fruit becoming even more tasteless, and possibly toxic. We can identify fruits that have been treated with carbide. When tomatoes are uniformly red, or mangoes and papaws are uniformly orange, one could easily make out that carbide may have been used. Plantains can also be identified if the stem is dark green while the fruits are all yellow. The implementation of the idea behind quick ripening of raw fruit is to make more profits. For fast ripening, 100g of carbide is used per 50kg of fruit. The chemical is dissolved in a coconut shell or similar basin placed in an airtight container. When the chemicals are dissolved, they release acetylene gas and the fruits are then piled on top and kept in the container for a day. The next day the raw fruits have turned ripe.

Ethrel

Another alternative would be to use ethrel. Ethrel has many uses such as hastening the production of flowering in fruit trees, as well as quickening the ripening process. When applied to plants it is absorbed and broken into ethylene, which is a natural non-toxic substance. Ethrel is commonly used in Australia and India. A minimal amount of ethrel is diluted in water, and containers are placed around the room. The fruits are then stacked in the room, and sodium hydroxide is added to the mixture. All ventilation to the room is then blocked off, and the fruits will ripen in three to five days in the gas that is released. The gas that is released is ethylene, the natural ripening agent found in fruits. This substance ensures that there is a uniform ripening of the fruits; in addition, the fruits retain their flavor. But it was pointed out by researchers that in both methods, whether using calcium carbide or ethrel, the chemical should not touch the substance. So, you need to watch out and think twice when your health is on the line.

Tyramine

Tyramine is a natural substance formed from the breakdown of protein as food ages. It is found in aged, fermented, or spoiled foods. The longer a high-protein food ages, the greater the tyramine content. Aged cheeses have the highest levels of tyramine. Some foods contain bacterial enzymes that convert tyrosine (amino acid) to tyramine. A tyramine-free diet is prescribed for people who are sensitive to tyramine, such as migraine sufferers, or those taking prescription antidepressants (monoamine oxidase inhibitor, MAOI) such as phenelzine. Under normal circumstances, tyramine and dopamine are metabolized to their harmless metabolites by the enzyme monoamine oxidase (MAO). Drugs that inhibit MAO also inhibit the metabolism of tyramine and dopamine, leading to elevated levels of these substances in the bloodstream. Excessive levels of tyramine can cause symptoms such as headache, palpitations, nausea, vomiting, and hypertension (high blood pressure). To avoid tyramine, ask about ingredients at restaurants and read food labels. Anything aged, dried, fermented, salted, smoked, or pickled is suspect. Watch out especially for pepperoni and salami.

Foods high in tyramine include aged cheeses: blue, boursault, boursin, brick (natural), brie, Camembert, cheddar, colby, Emmenthaler, Gruyere, mozzarella, Parmesan, provolone, Romano, Roquefort, and Swiss. It can also be found in American cheese, gouda, processed cheese, sour cream, and yogurt. Alcoholic beverages should be avoided during a tyramine cleanse, especially ale, Chinati, distilled spirits, most draft beers (including some non-alcoholic beers), port wine, sherry, and vermouth. Meats and fish to avoid if you have sensitivity to tyramine include canned meats, caviar, commercial gravies or meat extracts, fermented (hard) sausages, bologna, pepperoni, salami, summer sausage, Genoa salami, unrefrigerated and fermented fish, game meat, liver (beef or chicken), meat tenderizer, pickled herring, and potentially spoiled meat, poultry, or fish. Salted or dried fish, such as herring and cod or shrimp paste, should also be avoided. Fruits and vegetables to avoid during a tyramine cleanse include avocados (especially if they are overripe), bananas (because they contain dopamine), bean curd, Chinese pea pods, Chinese vegetables, eggplant, overripe fava beans and overripe figs, green bean pods, Italian flat beans, raisins (permitted on diets not restricted in dopamine), red plums, sauerkraut, soybean products that been stored more than a week, spinach, and tomatoes. Also avoid yeast extracts such as marmite and vegemite. Rounding out the list of foods to avoid in order to avoid tyramine are bouillon and other soup cubes, breads or crackers containing cheese, caffeine (in coffee, tea, or colas), chocolate, phenyl ethylamine, protein extracts, soy sauce, and products which contain yeast.

Toxic effects of tyramine

The toxic effects of tyramine are often described as "the cheese effect," especially when tyramine-induced damage occurs as a result of the use of MAO inhibitors. Tyramine can increase blood pressure (increasing the risk of hypertension) by causing the release of catecholamines, especially in the presence of MAO inhibitor drugs. People with high levels of candida albicans (yeast) should avoid tyramine-containing foods. Some people suffer from food allergies due to tyramine, causing the release of histamine from mast cells leading to the allergic reaction. Tyramine can cause anxiety, mood swings, depression, migraines, or headaches by overstimulating the adrenal glands, resulting in the depletion of the body's norepinephrine reserves. Tyramine can cause over stimulation of the autonomic nervous system as well.

A Healthy Body

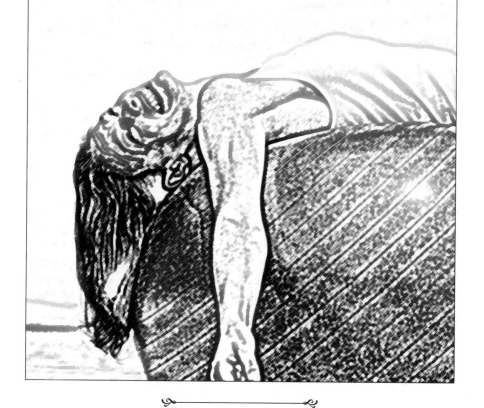

How can you protect your organs and have a healthy body?

To stay healthy, free of disease, and fit takes a lot of commitment from your side. Don't expect any quick fixes either. Looking for quick fixes only means you can be easily deceived by every person, and their products, which claim to have the magic solution for your health problems. This is especially true when it comes to weight loss, but applies to any disease.

I have learned from my professional experience that if you gain weight, it is the beginning of most disease processes, from diabetes to high cholesterol or even cancer. Now before you start on any diet or any program for losing weight, you should ask yourself — how did I end up here? Do not allow your emotions to be in charge of answering the question.

Every year in the United States people spend an estimated $34 billion on weight loss programs. It would be very surprising if anyone in this country was not aware of the war on fat. There has been increasing pressure in this country to lose weight. You can't read a newspaper, magazine, listen to the radio, or watch TV without being exposed to someone's latest idea of how to be thin. All the glory and rewards — money, friends, jobs, sex, health — are supposed to go to the thinnest people. Everything from sodas to breakfast cereals to cigarettes and magic peals are sold with the promise of weight loss. Like evangelists at the pulpit, the diet and medical industries tell us to shed those "extra pounds" or face the consequences. Who made thin in? All the chemicals and additives in your processed foods make you heavy. It is those same companies that also offer you great weight loss programs.

Among U.S. women 20 years and older, over 64 million are overweight, meaning their body mass index (BMI) is 25 to 29, while 34 million individuals with a BMI of 30 or more are considered obese.

Normal range for a female would be 15 to 25, depending on age and other factors. In 1990, there were 53 million dieters in the U.S. One survey found 62% of adults are dieting regularly and 18% are constantly on a diet.

In my practice, I have treated thousands of patients, and 75% of those patients tried every diet from NutriSystem, Jenny Craig, Atkins, South Beach, low carb, low fat, high protein, and vegetarian throughout their life. Food combining and many nutritional products, from prescription drugs to supplements, also claim to suppress the appetite or burn fat to lose weight and keep it off. So why do all these diets never work? That is the million-dollar question. If you knew the answer, then you could make a million.

As I mentioned before, every year in the U.S. people spend an estimated $34 billion on weight loss programs. When dieting, many problems can occur, from low energy and hunger to emotional highs and lows. Plus, during the diet, you are not losing the fat but rather you are losing water. When you get off the diet your weight comes back, plus more.

Your main concern should be your well-being and health, since nobody else cares, including your doctor. Insurance companies and pharmaceuticals develop medicines to relieve symptoms. It is in their interest to keep you on these medications. Some physicians get monetary bonuses for prescribing their drugs. They also might get other perks like fancy dinners and trips. Pharmaceuticals normally have one sales rep for every six doctors, which demonstrates how lucrative their relationship with the prescribing physician can be, so be a smart patient.

Not only do pharmaceutical companies not have your best interest at heart, food manufacturers are also not very concerned about their customers. Our overfed nation suffers from poor nourishment. In this country, the majority of the foods we eat are highly processed using refined sugar and are depleted of all nutrients, naturally occurring enzymes, fiber, vitamins, and minerals. Recently I was watching a news program. The reporter interviewed a mother in a rundown neighborhood in Chicago. She said it was easier to get a handgun or drugs than it was to get fresh vegetables and fruits in her neighborhood. Many studies have shown that the proper nutrients in a child's diet may help prevent or even reverse ADD, childhood obesity, and other common childhood diseases.

In this country our children do not eat a proper breakfast, if they eat anything at all. Our children are consuming fast food, cold cereals, and frozen food they pop in the microwave or in the toaster. These types of foods contain no enzymes and are full of sugar and empty nutrients, not to mention all the chemicals used for processing.

Soybeans

Ten percent of the cooking oil used in this country comes from soybeans. Soybeans have omega-6, which is an essential fatty acid our body needs in small amounts. An excess of omega-6 will deplete our omega-3, which is important for our overall health, especially for the brain. The worst by far is baby formula, which contains a lot of soy because it's usually the only food moms feed their babies as nourishment or as a substitution for mother's own milk. Soy contains phytoestrogens that can disrupt the baby's thyroid. The result of this disruption can cause asthma, allergies, and gastrointestinal damage, which decreases mineral absorption and can increase toxic levels of manganese that can cause neurological and brain damage associated with ADD/ADHD. Mothers should breast-fed at least for the first year. In Asia soy formula is traditionally not used for babies; the result is less childhood disease.

Soybeans contain a phytochemical known as isoflavones. Isoflavones are the compounds which are being studied in relation to the relief of certain menopausal symptoms, cancer prevention, slowing or reversing osteoporosis, and reducing the risk of heart disease. Soybeans, in their natural state, are not suitable for human consumption. Only after fermentation and extensive processing and extractions of certain chemicals in high temperatures do soybeans become good for us in moderation.

Soybeans contain a higher level of "phytic acid" than any other legume. Phytic acid can block the absorption of calcium, magnesium, iron, and zinc. Soybeans also contain potent enzyme-inhibitors, which block uptake of trypsin, which our bodies need for the digestion of protein (which can lead to deficiencies of amino acid in our bodies). In addition, soybeans also contain hemagglutinin, a clot-promoting substance that causes red blood cells to clump together. Hemagglutinin can be removed by fermentation in high temperatures.

Although Asia grows a whole lot of soybeans, it is not a main component of their food staples. In western society food processing companies do use a lot of soy. It is cheap. These companies separate the soybean into two categories, protein and oil. High-tech processing methods fail to remove the anti-nutrients and toxins that are naturally present in soybeans. The toxins of soy protein products are protein isolate, soy protein concentrate, texturized vegetable protein, and hydrolyzed vegetable protein. You will find these on the ingredient label in many processed and packaged foods such as protein powders, milk shakes, energy bars, baked goods, crackers, canned foods, french fries, frozen foods, and veggie burgers. The worst soy oil products are margarines and shortenings made from partially hydrogenated soybean oil containing dangerous trans fatty acids. Most of the liquid vegetable oils sold in supermarkets also come from the soybean. Look on page 148 for a list of healthy cooking oils.

A Quick Detour
Changing your health means changing your mind

Congratulations, you care enough about your health to have made it this far into the book. Now you are going to start reading about what you need to do to help yourself, specific instructions starting with the chapter on the components of optimum health and weight. To do what you need to do your head has to be in the right place and you will need to maintain that mind-set.

Ask yourself . . . Do you ever feel like a robot, programed to get an impossibly long list of mind numbing work done. By the time you make it home the only thing you want to do is fall on the couch in front of the TV. Perhaps you'll indulge in a glass of wine to stunt your busy mind so that you can fall into a restless sleep.

Cook a healthy dinner? Forget it. Take a walk? To tired. Get up early to go to the gym? No time, you have an early morning meeting, or perhaps you are dropping the kids off at school. There is always an excuse.

That's right, excuse. No one is at their optimum health if they don't start with their head. Changing your mind and making yourself a priority is the number one criteria for getting healthy.

All those people you believe depend on you, well what will they do after you are gone. Stop worrying about the Jones's and start worrying about yourself.

A rut is a hard place to escape from. It requires you to commit a selfish act and make your health a priority. You don't have to go cold turkey. You can start in small ways. Why not walk at home instead of health club to save precious time. Why not choose only fresh and naturally food at the grocery store so that you don't have

---

Look at the diagram to the right.
Do you feel any of the emotions
on the outside of the large triangle.

If you picked one, the bad news
is you have all three.
They are inseparable.
They form what I term
the triangle of death.

Inside this triangle
are symptoms that come
with these emotions
and you are in the
center.

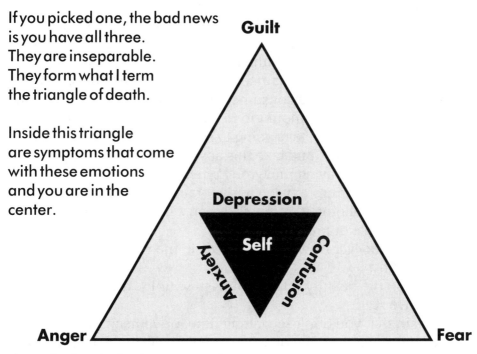

If you feel guilt, forgive yourself.
If you feel fear, face it.
If you feel anger, walk away.

Achieve this and you will have won!

---

any temptations at home. Park the car a little further away so you get an extra bit of walking in. Play ball with the kids instead of watching a video together. Take the dog for a walk.

I tell many of my patients to sit down a write a list from one to ten of their priorities for themselves. This is an exercise in changing mind set. You have to know where you are going before you plan how to get there. Ask yourself what is your purpose in life. I bet your answer will not include the word robot, or the phrases "rush hour," or "work myself to death."

Like a robot, the battery has died. When your energy is low ("I don't have time for breakfast) your brain doesn't work. You find the time to take your car in for a tune up, but what about yourself.

It is criminal the way so many of us treat our body. The stress, the sugar, the poisons that we consume, and the way we use food as an emotional switch is tantamount to needing a good psychiatrist.

Save the time you will take going to see a counselor about why you are killing yourself and take this advice instead.

- When you are craving the wrong types of food take 3 deep breaths. This brings oxygen to the brain. Then drink a glass of water, and walk for 10 minutes. If you still want that candy, eat a good source of protein instead.
- Divorce whoever or whatever stands in the way of your quest to get healthy.
- Focus on the healthy relationships in your life and let go of the negative stuff.
- Explain that you don't see taking time for yourself as a selfish act, but rather a giving one, because you will be better able to help those around you when you are energized and feeling good.
- Ask yourself, am I really hungry or is something else going on.

Components of optimum health and weight

Consume organically grown food

Diet plays an important role in health and disease. The foods we choose can help in the prevention of many illnesses, thus increasing the quality of life. More than ever before, many people are choosing organic foods over conventionally grown foods containing synthetic fertilizers or pesticides that seep into fruits and vegetables beyond the skin. The chemicals that have been used on farms are strong enough to kill insects and plant infections. They can also be harmful to the human body and environment.

In this country there are literally hundreds of permitted pesticides, herbicides, insecticides, fungicides, hormones, antibiotics, and other chemical additives present in non-organic food — not to mention other additives and flavorings that have been added after cultivation and during food processing. Over 3,000 high-risk toxins are present in the U.S. food supply, which by law are excluded from organic foods. These include 73 pesticides classified by the Environmental Protection Agency as potential carcinogens. Our water supply also has been contaminated with these chemicals. Organically grown food must be watered with spring water and so is not subject to the same contaminations — more reasons for us to eat organic food. Organic foods we should eat include fruits, vegetables, grains, eggs, and dairy, meats, and poultry in moderation. We hear so often "you are what you eat." Fruits and veggies grown organically show significantly higher levels of cancer-fighting antioxidants.

Foods that should be eaten organically

▸ Baby food — According to the National Academy of Sciences, federal pesticide standards provide too little health protection.

▸ Strawberries — A 1993 study by the Environmental Working Group found that supermarket strawberries were the most heavily contaminated fruit or vegetable in the U.S.

▸ Rice — Water-soluble herbicides and insecticides have contaminated the groundwater near rice fields. Buy organic wild rice and brown rice.

▸ Oats — In 1994, the FDA found illegal residues in a year's worth of Cheerios manufactured by General Mills. Organic growers provide oats, millet, quinoa, barley, couscous, amaranth, and spelt as healthy options. Use organic steel-cut oats.

▸ Milk — Dairy companies inject cows with recombinant bovine growth hormone. Seventy-nine percent of treated cows get clinical mastitis, a common udder infection. Treating them with antibiotics increases the chance of antibiotic residue in milk. Another toxic aspect of milk is xanthine oxidase, which would normally be rejected by your body, but homogenization causes the human digestive system to absorb it. This means you are absorbing molybdenum, an enzyme of bovine milk. This enzyme will clog your arteries, cause premature aging, cause free radicals, and increase your chance for gout by increasing uric acid. Do not consume milk; if you do, choose organic milk, which is widely available.

▸ Bell peppers — The FDA found that in 1993, 38% of the peppers from Mexico, which provides 98% of the U.S. supply, had two or more toxic pesticides within the pepper.

▸ Bananas — Costa Rica uses 35% of the country's pesticide

on banana crops. This pesticide is not sprayed, but rather is absorbed.

▶ Green beans — Sixty pesticides are used on green beans. Ten percent of Mexican green beans are contaminated with pesticides that are illegal in the U.S.

▶ Peaches — The FDA cited peaches for above-average rates of illegal pesticide violations; 5% of the crop was contaminated.

▶ Nuts — Because of the high fat content, they hold on to pesticides more than others types of crops.

▶ Anything your kids eat more than three times a week. Using organic foods will lessen the accumulation of pesticides in their bodies.

Other highly contaminated foods, according to some sources, that should be eaten organically are spinach, cherries (grown in the U.S.), cantaloupe (grown in Mexico), celery, apples, apricots, grapes (grown in Chile), and cucumbers.

According to some researchers, who have been funded by interest groups, eating organically grown food puts consumers at risk of the following diseases: food poisoning from salmonella, E.coli, cryptosporidiosis, and mycotoxin poisoning. Their reasoning is that organic farmers use animal wastes as fertilizer. Animal manure is a reservoir of enteric pathogens. If this were true, then my family and I should be very sick, since we have been eating organically grown food for the past 10 years.

Prepare your own food

Preparing your own food has many advantages:

▶ Safety and peace of mind
▶ Freshness
▶ Cost

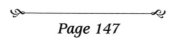

Commercially processed foods contain additional fat, salt, sugar, fillers, or other ingredients that are completely unnecessary for good nutrition. These additives are an attempt to add flavor, texture, and bulk to poor-quality products. They contribute nothing at all to our health or well-being. By preparing your own food, you can be sure that you are getting complete nutrients, plus freshness and less contamination from your food. Even preparing your baby food or your dog food is a good idea. Consider what you have read or heard about all the recalls of dog food. If you make the choice to prepare homemade dog food, you can control everything that your dog eats. You can feed him nutritious food that includes vegetables, rice, liver, and lean meats. Cooking for your dog means you help him stay healthy and free of disease. The choice is in your hands. If you don't know how to cook, start to learn. It could be a great adventure.

Use the right type of oil

The best oils for cooking and frying are those that have a high smoking point, which means they can be heated to high temperatures before burning.

Coconut oil

Coconut oil is commonly used in manufacturing baked goods, especially when frying. It has a high smoke point of 170°C (350°F). Extra virgin coconut oil is good for this purpose. The health benefits of coconut oil include lauric acid — found in mother's milk! Lauric acid is the predominant type of medium chain saturated fatty acid that turns into a substance called monolaurin. This is the actual compound responsible for helping to strengthen the immune system. It promotes good heart health, weight loss, and supports your immune system by increasing metabolism. Coconut oil is a good source of immediate energy.

Olive oil

Cooking with olive oil is like cooking with wine. Never use a wine or olive oil that does not taste good to you. Olives are fruit and olive oil is a juice of that fruit. Olive oil will turn rancid when exposed to air, heat, and light. If your oil's taste changes to a buttery taste, then it's probably rancid. The ideal temperature for storing olive oil is 57°F (14°C), although it works very well at a room temperature of 70°F. Olive oil should be stored in a dark area where the temperature remains fairly constant. Extra virgin olive oil is great for salad dressing, dipping your bread, and to top off your potatoes. It is also great on cooked vegetables and rice. Use olive oil when you saute food on low heat, as long as the color of oil doesn't change.

Grape seed oil

Grape seed oil is great for cooking or frying, is light and medium-yellow to green color, is an aromatic oil, and is a by-product of wine making. It is used in salads and some cooking. Its smoking point is 420°F (216 °C). Grape seed oil improves HDL cholesterol due to omega-3 (A-linolenic acid), omega-6 (linoleic acid), and omega-9 (oleic acid).

Eat your meals in balance

Are you always on the run in an unbalanced life? Do you never seem to have quite enough time in the day? Sound familiar?

Lack of time is a major reason why many people give up eating right. They probably are not thinking about their next meal, or if they do think of it, it is usually not a healthy choice. Time is money, as they say, which is one of the reasons our car has become our dining table. In fact, healthy eating is now more prevalent in the books we read or the TV shows we watch than in our kitchen.

When prioritizing your daily schedule, make what and when you are going to eat number one. When you have a good diet, it helps your body withstand stress and provides the energy necessary to make it through the day.

Eating smaller meals also is a great idea for your health. Digesting a large meal takes more energy than you use to circulate the blood through your body, running your respiratory system — even more that some exercise.

When digesting our food, the first step is creating acid in the stomach. In order to digest our food, we secrete the right amount of hydrochloric acid, a strong mineral acid produced by the parietal cells of the stomach.

Hydrochloric acid is comprised of 0.2% - 0.5% of gastric juice, as well as other enzymes needed for digestion, like pancreatic enzymes. Since each and every enzyme must be made by the body from scratch, it takes a lot of chemical energy to make the enzymes we need to digest our food. By eating small meals, we will not be stressing our energy supply and stressing the organ which produces those enzymes.

The other reason for eating smaller, more frequent meals has to do with calories. The body has to process the food into energy for immediate use. If we don't burn up the calories in a reasonable amount of time, those calories will eventually become fat cells. Also, eating frequent and smaller meals prevents the ups and downs of your blood sugar level. Letting your insulin production look like a roller coaster means you could become insulin resistant, which will lead to obesity and diabetes. I highly suggest people over 40 who have enzyme insufficiencies should take digestive enzymes.

Eat the right type of fat

Fat is needed for your body to function properly. Fat is used as an energy source. Cholecystokinin (CCK), a hormone that is released when you eat fatty food, suppresses the appetite. It provides a sense of fullness after meals.

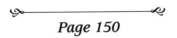

Fat is used in several hormone-like compounds called eicosanoids. These compounds help protect vital organs and regulate blood pressure, heart rate, blood vessel constriction, blood clotting, healthy hair and skin, and the nervous system. Also, dietary fat carries fat-soluble vitamins — vitamins A, D, E, and K — from your food into your liver.

Healthy fats

Choosing the right type of fats can affect your health; your best options are monounsaturated and polyunsaturated fats. These fats can lower your risk of heart disease by reducing the total cholesterol and low-density lipoprotein (LDL) levels in your blood. The cholesterol component of our cells also is the main substance in fatty deposits (plaques) that can develop in our arteries. Plaques that build up in arteries can reduce blood flow through our vessels, which increases the risk of heart disease and stroke.

Types of good fat

Polyunsaturated fats like omega-3, which are found mostly in seafood, are good.

Sources of omega-3 fatty acids include cold-water fish, such as salmon and mackerel, and herring, which is especially beneficial to the heart. Omega-3s appear to decrease the risk of coronary artery disease.

Flaxseeds, flax oil, and walnuts also contain omega-3 fatty acids and small amounts are found in soybean and canola oils. Polyunsaturated fats, which you should avoid, include vegetable oils such as safflower, corn, sunflower, soy, and cottonseed oils. Monounsaturated fats include olive, peanut, and canola

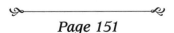

oils. Avocados and most nuts also have high amounts of monounsaturated fat. Your best choice is olive oil; try to avoid peanut and canola oils. Most of these fats are liquid at room temperature.

Fats you should avoid

We also should know too much fat can have a negative impact on your health. Like any other food, eating large amounts of high-fat foods, such as saturated fat or trans fat, adds excess calories, which can lead to weight gain and obesity. Obesity is an increased risk factor for several diseases, including diabetes, high cholesterol, coronary artery, heart disease, cancer, gallstones, osteoarthritis, and varicose veins.

Saturated fat, usually solid at room temperature, is most often found in animal products — such as red meat, poultry, butter, and whole milk. Other foods high in saturated fat include coconut, palm, and other tropical oils. Read about coconut oil in another part of this chapter.

Trans fatty acids

Trans fat comes from adding hydrogen to vegetable oil through a process called hydrogenation. This makes the fat more solid and less likely to turn rancid. Hydrogenated fat is a common ingredient in commercial baked goods (junk food) such as doughnuts, french fries, crackers, cookies, and cakes. Shortenings and margarines also are high in trans fat. As of January 2006, food manufacturers are required to list trans fat content on nutrition labels. Amounts less than 0.5 grams per serving are listed as 0 grams trans fat on the food label.

Have your daily protein

Surprisingly little is known about protein and health. The body needs protein every day to build and repair muscles and other body

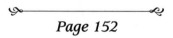

tissues, to make hormones, and to make enzymes speed up and help certain chemical reactions to occur in the body.

According to the RDA, adults need a minimum of 0.8 grams of protein for every kilogram of body weight per day to keep from slowly breaking down their own tissues. Muscles are built from protein. Unlike fat cells for fat and glucose stored in muscles or in the liver, there is no place in the body to store protein. We need to consume sufficient protein daily to allow our muscles to be healthy and perform at their peak. Food protein is classified in two groups — complete and incomplete. Complete protein comes from animal sources like fish, chicken, dairy, beef, and so on. Incomplete protein comes from legumes, nuts, seeds, and vegetables. Plant protein is absorbed at about 70-90%, animal protein at 85-100%. There is concern among some that plant protein will not provide enough protein alone. This is not a problem in this country (North America), where presently we eat two to three times the RDA for animal protein anyway. Consumption of four to six ounces of good protein daily is necessary for good health. On the other hand, consuming too much protein increases the body's water requirement and may contribute to dehydration, because the kidneys require more water to eliminate the excess nitrogen load of a high protein intake.

Eat the right type of complex carbohydrates

Complex carbohydrates, or polysaccharides, are made mostly of long strands of simple sugars. They are found in fruits, grains, nuts, seeds, legumes, and vegetables. The best sources of carbohydrates are grain products (preferably whole grains) such as bread, brown rice, cereal, and pasta, as well as fruits and vegetables. Food labels tell you how many grams of total carbohydrates are in a serving of that food. All grains contain complex carbohydrates; however, whole grains — such as whole wheat pasta — are better for you because they have more fiber. Carbohydrates are important to replenish and maintain glycogen store. Each day, the endurance athlete should try to eat at least 15 servings of complex carbohydrate products, at least six servings of fruits, and six servings of vegetables.

Breakfast is the most important meal of the day

You remember being encouraged to eat breakfast, especially by mom, and you know mom is always right. Breakfast is important for all ages. Other studies show a connection between skipping breakfast with weight gain and memory impairment in young and older adults. When parents do not eat breakfast, how can they expect their children to eat breakfast? Start your day with whole grains, eggs, and fruits. A good high-fiber breakfast will fill you up and help maintain your energy, mental performance, memory, and mood during the active part of your day.

Low glycemic index diet

The glycemic index relates to the way your body's sugar levels respond to certain foods. Foods are given a rating from 0 to100 on the glycemic index (from artichoke at 15 to cherries at 22 to sweet potato at 54), with glucose (sugar) in the highest position. High glycemic index foods (such as simple carbohydrates) will increase the body's sugar levels rapidly, whereas low glycemic index foods will increase the body's sugar levels slowly. A good understanding of the glycemic index can assist in weight loss and help control diabetes. Eat foods with glycemic indexes less than 45, which produce a small rise in blood sugar and insulin levels. Foods with low glycemic indexes are vegetables, legumes, fruits, grains (complex carbohydrate), nuts, and proteins.

Drink warm water with one-half teaspoon of fresh lemon juice half an hour before your breakfast.

Lemon water is tasty, refreshing, and best of all, in the morning it eliminates water retention and helps with weight reduction, plus keeps the system alkaline. Lemon is extremely alkaline and raises the water's alkalinity. During the night when we sleep, the body's acidity rises; by drinking the warm lemon water first thing in the morning, we bring the body pH to alkaline. Apart from being an amazing body alkalizer, lemon water also has the following health benefits:

▶▶ Lemons are antiseptic.

▶▶ Lemon water has excellent digestive properties to ease heartburn, bloating, and other digestion problems.

▶▶ Lemon water stimulates and cleanses the liver.

▶▶ Lemon water stimulates and cleanses the kidneys.

▶▶ Lemon water is a great skin cleanser.

▶▶ Lemon water provides relief for cold and flu symptoms by boosting the immune system.

Don't drink liquid 15 minutes before and 30 minutes after your meals.

Drinking liquids (even water) with your meal will affect your digestion by decreasing or diluting the acid of your stomach, which slows down the digestion, perhaps causing indigestion, bloating, and weight gain.

Combine foods wisely

Let's talk about eating a pepperoni pizza. You have two proteins, a carbohydrate and a fat, all at the same time. Different types of food require different digestive enzyme secretions. When I eat pizza all the necessary enzymes secrete. The problem with this is that the digestive system slows down because these foods digest at different rates. Eat most of your carbohydrates in the morning, because this is an energy source. Avoid milk or dairy products with other proteins and sugar. Try for zero carbs at dinner time because carbs cause an influx of insulin.

No chewing gum

Secretion of acid and enzymes for digestion starts with our vision when we see the food, or with our nose when we smell the food, or when we taste food, or when we chew our food. Chewing is important to break down the food and cause secretion of acid.

The majority of people will chew gum on an empty stomach, which causes damage to the stomach cell because the cell eventually will stop secreting when it has been overworked. This causes hypochlorhydria (low acid in stomach). Hypochlorhydria may cause low thyroid function, which in turn affects metabolism.

Gum typically contains a sweetener of some type. Chewing gum that contains sugar can be harmful to your teeth. Sugar fuels the acid-producing bacteria in your mouth. Most chewing gum contains aspartame. Many medical experts have found that the amount of aspartame in chewing gum and other products can lead to numerous side effects, from headaches to seizures and much more. Aspartame at 86°F (remember the body temperature is 98.6°F) turns to formaldehyde, commonly attributed to damage to the cells and organs.

Twenty minutes of daily relaxation

Walking is one of the best, safest, and most natural forms of relaxation. Walk in a relaxed way, but with good posture, shoulders down, arms swinging naturally as you walk; in fact, you can walk any time, any place. Walking also is effective exercise for people of all ages and all states and levels of health. What's more, walking increases our sense of well-being. Think about it — walking 20 minutes every day after work or before meals will help decrease stress and balance well-being before sitting at the table to add nutrients to the body.

Fresh fruits and vegetables daily

We should eat at least five servings of fruits and three servings of vegetables (organically grown) daily. Fruits and vegetables are great for better health and more servings are even better.

Juicing is the best way to achieve the most nutrients.

Eating a diet rich in fruits and vegetables may reduce the risk of cardiovascular diseases and type 2 diabetes, protect against certain cancers (mouth, stomach, and colon-rectum cancer), and also reduce the risk of developing kidney stones and osteoporosis. Vegetables are low in calories and can be substituted for high calorie food for maintaining healthy weight. Juicing raw fruits and vegetables is one of the best ways to get the maximum benefit from these foods. The important point is that the juice is fresh and in its raw, natural state, which has the highest level of nutrients, antioxidants, and live enzymes, so the body can quickly absorb larger amounts of nutrients. The best juice is your own, rather than buying the prepackaged juice from the supermarket.

Chew your food at least 25 times

Chewing is the first step of the digestive process, called mastication. Mastication means what we put in our mouth is ground up into smaller pieces and mixed with some digestive enzymes, called amylase, which our saliva produces to begin the digestive process. Our digestion will extract beneficial minerals and vitamins from what we eat and expel the rest. This process involves breaking down our food into smaller and smaller pieces. When some of those pieces are small enough, they are absorbed into your bloodstream. Other components, like insoluble fiber, continue on through your intestines and help to expel other waste products and to clean the surfaces of our intestines. When we do not properly chew our food, what we have eaten will go through our digestive system as large pieces. Our bodies do not have teeth anywhere else. After we swallow our food, there is no other place in our bodies to break up large pieces of food. The acid from the stomach and the enzymes from the pancreas, then to the small intestine, will only be able to act on the exposed surfaces of the food. Chewing properly is the only way to grind up food so that it is small enough to allow the rest of the digestive system to extract all the nutrients from the broken food as much as possible. Also, when you take a bite, chew it 25 times before swallowing; most people chew their food about 10 times. If you increase each bite to 25 times, you will notice how much more flavor you register, along with how much more satisfied your feel after a meal. Take a rest between each bite and eat slower. You will find that you eat less and get satisfied more quickly. This way of eating will help control your weight, and you may even lose weight.

Food portions and servings

You remember mom said cleaning your plate is good? Not any more. In this country people are confused about normal servings. Everything is served or sold as large packages, and often times that becomes normal and so we eat without paying attention to how much we are eating. Most of the food we eat has been enhanced with more flavors to make it tastier, so that we eat more. We always get better deals on larger packages, and we wonder why we are getting fatter by the day. Obesity in this country has increased as portion sizes have grown in this country. Twenty years ago, a basic meal at a fast-food restaurant consisted of a small burger, with cheese or without, small fries, and an 8-ounce soft drink. Today, your order may include a double- or triple-patty burger with extra cheese, "super sized" fries, and a 20-ounce soda. We can improve portion size by learning to better judge the amount of food on our plate or serving bowl. Some research shows that the more food we have on hand, the more we will eat.

Keep the body on the alkaline side

When your body becomes acidic, you become more prone to disease. All biochemical reactions and electrical (life) energy are under pH control. Excess acidity in the body causes all sorts of degenerative diseases including arthritis, cancer, gall stones, heart disease, kidney stones, osteoporosis, and more.

An acid pH is hot and fast, like the battery of your car, an acid battery. On cold days you want your car to start fast.

An alkaline pH, on the other hand, biochemically speaking, is slow and cool, like an alkaline battery in a flashlight. You want that battery to be cool and to burn out slowly.

The body has a homeostatic mechanism that maintains a constant pH of 7.4 in the blood. This mechanism works by depositing and withdrawing acid and alkaline minerals from other locations, including the bones, soft tissues, body fluids, and saliva. Therefore, the pH of these other tissues can fluctuate greatly.

One test we can perform is checking the pH in saliva. Saliva offers a window through which we can see the overall pH balance in the body. Most diseases cannot exist in an alkaline environment, like cancer and arthritis. All forms of arthritis are associated with excess acidity.

The body's pH is very important because pH controls the speed of the body's biochemical reactions by controlling the speed of enzyme activity, as well as the speed that electricity moves through the body. The higher the alkalinity of a substance or solution, the more electrical resistance that substance or solution holds. Therefore, in higher pH, electricity travels slower. When the body is more acidic, we are more exhausted, burned out, and we are prone to anger quicker. In this society we are running hot and fast, and to answer the question of how we got there, we don't have to look

(Continued page 161)

Criteria for the right supplements

The FDA will allow supplemental manufacturers to show an HVL's designation on their products if their manufacturing practices and procedures are designed to monitor and verify quality throughout every step of the production process. These processes include:

▶▶ Current Good Manufacturing Practices — cGMPs for nutritional supplements in accordance with USP27 (US Pharmacopoeia) are followed.
▶▶ SOPs are written in accordance with cGMP27.
▶▶ Three in-house laboratories to ensure product quality under the supervision of staff PhDs, to ensure product quality and consistency.
▶▶ Laboratories test for chemical analysis — ensuring potency of formula components.
▶▶ Laboratories tests for physical analysis — ensuring dosage weight, hardness, disintegration, and overall consistency and appearance.
▶▶ Laboratories test for microbiology — ensuring all raw materials and products do not contain yeast, mold, or bacterial impurities in accordance with USP27.
▶▶ HVL tests all raw materials for the following: microbiological contamination, authenticity, potency, heavy metals, chemical solvents, peroxides and anisidines (markers for rancidity), pesticides, and dioxins (PCBs).
▶▶ HVL laboratories are ISO 9001 certified and ISO 17025 accredited. These standards mean that HVL is compliant with one of the highest and most recognized standards of quality in the world. It means conformance to a global standard that is independent of industry influences. It also demonstrates a tangible commitment to quality that is internationally understood and accepted. Very few manufacturers of nutritional supplements in the world have ISO 17025 accreditation.
▶▶ HVL is FDA audit compliant.
▶▶ HVL meets Bioterrorism compliance for published requirements for all raw materials incorporated into their nutritional supplements.

So whenever you purchase a dietary supplement or vitamin, look for HVL accredited on the label. Be sure to purchase capsules and not tablets; capsules are easier on the digestive system and don't contain fillers.

far. First start with our food. In the morning we start breakfast with coffee (acid) and donuts (acid), then lunch is fast food or boxed food (acid), with the drink being colas (acid), and at dinner time we finish with pizza (acid). Violence has increased as the number of fast food restaurants have increased. Watch what you put in your mouth. The general "rule of thumb" is to eat 20% acidic foods and 80% alkaline foods. It is hard to completely avoid acidic foods.

Strongly acidic food: meats, dairy
Mildly acidic food: grains, nuts
Mildly alkaline food: vegetables, fruits, berries
Strongly alkaline food: supplements
(calcium, magnesium, potassium)
Fats and oils have a neutral pH

Use the right supplements

With the passage of the Dietary Supplement Health and Education Act (DSHEA) in 1994, the public has been more easily able to purchase a wide variety of herbs, vitamins, minerals, and other ingredients to support optimal health and supplement the nutrients that may be absent from their diet. However, in the years since the passage, there has been a great deal of confusion surrounding the dietary supplement industry, especially in regards to quality, safety, and accountability.

Dietary supplements are not drugs or over-the-counter medications; however, the Food and Drug Administration (FDA) has some regulatory rules regarding the manufacture of vitamins and supplements. The FDA maintains important regulatory authority, including the ability to remove unsafe products from the marketplace, as well as overseeing which ingredients can be sold legally as supplements. The FDA also monitors claims that are made about dietary supplements, as these claims cannot include statements about treating or curing a disease. If such a claim is made, the product can be defined as a drug and the FDA has the authority to take enforcement action. One important topic to note — the U.S. government oversees manufacturing practices and procedures designed to monitor and verify quality throughout every step of the production process of supplements. Our supplements are also subject to the same rigorous safety procedures.

Daily sunlight for 30 minutes between 9-10am or 4-5pm

These times are suggested because there will be less UV damage to the skin. I suggest to my patients here in the Northwest that they take 2000 IU of vitamin D3 daily.

Sun affects our bodies and releases chemicals in the brain that affect our mood. Sunlight, like exercise, is a factor in our health, although you have to remember too much sunshine can have very adverse effects on your overall health, due to ultraviolet rays. Bone loss due to inadequate vitamin D formation in the skin also occurs in people exposed only to ordinary indoor light. Vitamin D, most of which results from exposure to the sun's ultraviolet rays, is needed to absorb calcium from the diet, and many people in northern latitudes become deficient in vitamin D during the winter. The problem is most serious among those who spend the daylight hours indoors, and foods fortified with vitamin D are not always adequate compensation. Different parts of the spectrum have different effects. While the invisible ultraviolet is needed for vitamin D synthesis and sun tanning, the visible part of the spectrum influences body rhythms and hormone levels. Light exerts its internal biochemical effects through the eye. Light passes through the retina to the optic nerve. Part of the optic nerve goes to the brain's vision center and the other part goes to a section of the hypothalamus, the suprachiasmatic nucleus, which is the body's internal clock. From this nucleus, the light-generated nerve message travels through the brain to the spinal cord and out a nerve center, called the superior cervical ganglion, which transmits it to the pineal gland.

Use of a sauna two times a month

I advised you consult your physician before breaking a sweat. Saunas are hazardous to individuals with high or low blood pressure and heart disease, and individuals under the influence of alcohol or drugs and pregnant women should avoid saunas. Don't take a sauna when you are ill, and if you feel unwell during your sauna, step out. Use of a sauna for 10-15 minutes will increase your heart rate up to 75%. The result is the same as physical exercise and increased cardiac load, equivalent to a brisk walk.

Heat also causes blood vessels in skin to expand and become more flexible and increases circulation to the extremities, which brings nutrients to subcutaneous and surface tissue. Skin is the biggest organ in our body; 30% of our body wastes or toxins are passed through the skin. Profuse sweating enhances the detoxifying, which results in a healthy body and healthy skin. Body temperature rises during a sauna to 40°C (104°F), and internal body temperature can rise to 38°C (100.4°F). High heat from the sauna creates an artificial fever in the body. Fever stimulates the immune system by increasing white blood cells, antibodies, and interferon, resulting in the fighting of disease. Detoxing also helps to reduce cellulite and relieves the pain and stiffness of arthritis. Drinking two to four glasses of cool water during and after each sauna is necessary to replace your water loss during your sauna. Use of a dry sauna keeps the humidity at about 20%. Just don't keep it too dry or you might experience respiratory difficulties. Our bodies tolerate dry heat better than a wet sauna.

You can also use an infrared sauna. Infrared saunas work using infrared heaters to convert light directly to heat. This heat has the effect of warming nearby objects without raising the air temperature, which people can tolerate better than a regular sauna.

Bowel movements and urination

Bowel movements one to three times daily are normal, but it all depends on what we eat and how much we eat. An average healthy person should have at least one to two bowel movements per day in order to keep their system clean and free of diseases. Bowel movements should be formed and long and be free of undigested food. Time sitting on the toilet should be less than three minutes. If you stay there over 5-10 minutes pushing, straining, or paining to have a bowel movement, then you are constipated.

▶▶ Bowl movements 1-3 times daily.
▶▶ Bowl movements should be formed.
▶▶ Bowl movements should be free of undigested food.

The average urine output for adults is 1.5 liters (six cups) a day and that can increase, depending on water intake (urination should equal three-fourths of water intake). When you experience excess urination, thirst, and hunger, consult with your doctor.

Use of water

The internal temperature of the body is controlled with water. Water makes up to 92% of the blood in the body and nearly 98% of intestinal, gastric, saliva, and pancreatic juices. Cartilage is composed of 65 to 85% water. Muscles are composed of 70 to 75% water. Water comprises 10% of the body's adipose tissue (fat cells) and water comprises 70% of the dermis of the skin (which represents 15 to 18% of the total water content of the body). Water holds all nutritive factors in solution and acts as a transportation medium to the various parts of the body for these substances. The mucous membranes need plenty of water to keep them soft and free from friction on their delicate surfaces. Another important function of water is to flush the toxins and salt from the body, like taking a shower to clean the outside of the body every day. Water irrigates and cleanses the kidneys and acts as a carrier vehicle for the kidneys' excretion of toxins from the body. Drinking the right kind (filtered) and amount of water will help with better circulation, which is most important for optimum health and a long life. When we substitute water with other types of liquids like alcohol, tea, coffee, and cola drinks, it increases toxins, which causes damage to all organs and cells. Water is the most important component for our health. We should not become dehydrated. Many of us have a dehydrated appearance with symptoms such as parched, leathery, or dry skin. Wrinkles may appear on our foreheads and around the eyes. Another sign of dehydration is constipation. Long-term water deficiency (dehydration) is a contributing factor in some cases of hypertension. If you feel thirsty, you are already dehydrated. Alcoholic beverages and caffeinated drinks both increase urine output and make you become more dehydrated.

If you experience symptoms such as cramping muscles and feeling faint, and do not begin to feel better once you have gotten out of the heat and had some water or sports-type drink, you should contact your physician. If you are experiencing symptoms of severe dehydration, which include loss of consciousness and little or no urination, you need to seek medical attention immediately.

Do not drink tap water.

Tap water may be contaminated with these substances:

DDT

Aldrin

Dieldrin

Carbon tetrachloride

Tap water is sometimes contaminated with arsenic and prone to contamination with lead (from water pipes).

Excessive consumption of water causes excretion of pangamic

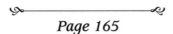

acid, choline, folic acid, inositol, para aminobenzoic acid (PABA), and vitamin C.

Use filtered water for showering

Chlorine is added to all municipal water supplies. This disinfectant hardens arteries, destroys proteins in the body, and irritates skin and sinuses. When you take a shower, chlorine (at 140°F) turns to chloroform. This powerful by-product of chlorination causes excessive free radical formation (accelerated aging!), causes normal cells to mutate, and cholesterol to oxidize, which increases LDL. It is a known carcinogen. People with allergies, asthma, and respiratory problems should avoid showering with chlorinated water. You should use filtered water for washing your fruits and vegetables and for cooking, or for anything else you consume.

Cookwear

Cast iron

Cast iron cooking has been with us for thousands of years, going back to ancient China. Cast iron is excellent for browning, frying, stewing, and baking foods. Today's cast iron is made of iron alloys that give additional strength. Prior to regular use, seal your cast iron (seasoning). Cooking in cast iron is known to greatly increase the dietary source of iron. This is true when cooking foods high in acid, such as tomato-based sauces. There is less of an effect for foods that are quickly fried in the skillet.

As you might expect, frequent stirring of food will also increase the amount of iron. Cooking in cast iron can often provide all of the iron that a body needs. Cast iron takes a while to heat; the advantage is, once heated, it will remain very hot for a long period of time. As such, foods that require high heat are best cooked in cast iron as it will not change the taste of your food. Store your cast iron cookware with the lids off, especially in humid weather. When covered, moisture can build up and cause rust. Should rust appear, the pan should be re-seasoned. After each wash, preheat your cast iron, causing it to dry before storing.

Stainless steel

Stainless steel is really a mixture of several different metals, including nickel, chromium, and molybdenum. If any minerals leak into the cooked food, it will only be minimal amounts. This type of pan is very strong and long lasting. It usually won't stain, tarnish, or corrode.

Avoid storing your hot food in plastic containers and using plastics utensils. (Hard plastics leak fewer chemicals than flexible ones.)

Use of glass or stainless steel is a good choice, even for water bottles, and try not to purchase any liquid food packaged in plastic.

Avoid use of microwave

Microwave cooking heats food from the center out, cooking the food very quickly. This causes foods to lose some of their nutrients. In addition to this, if you cook this food in plastic, it causes dioxin, which can get into the food. But worst of all is that most food cooked in the microwave is processed food from out of the freezer, something you shouldn't eat at all.

No lead, copper or aluminum

Use glass, porcelain, enamel, or terra cotta clay pans, which do not contain lead.

Use wooden bowls and wooden utensils (for salads); hard plastics leak fewer chemicals than flexible ones.

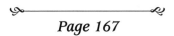

Don't use cookwear which contains copper (pots and pans, gelatin molds).

Don't use cookwear which contains aluminum (use stainless steel pots and pans). Popcorn wrappers (the kind you stick in the microwave) also contain aluminum. Aluminum foil should also not be used for cooking.

Excess aluminum stored in the brain can cause Alzheimer's disease.

Avoid products containing or wrapped with lead or cadmium.

The lining of a can, used to store or preserve food, often contains cadmium. Many processed foods such as candy and margarine also can contain cadmium. Wines are susceptible to lead contamination from the seals used in the bottling process. And don't forget that lead crystal that you might drink your wine out of. Some cosmetics and hair color products also contain lead. Interestingly, the ingestion of dairy products can increase absorption of lead in the body.

Lead exposure is still a public health problem in the United States.

Lead competes in the body with calcium, causing numerous malfunctions in calcium-facilitated cellular metabolism and calcium uptake and usage. It can inhibit neurotransmitters to blockade calcium channels. Lead will also affect the central nervous system.

Neurobehavioral deficits resembling attention deficit disorder (ADD) have also been found in lead-exposed children. Poor quality nutrition, including deficiencies in calcium and iron, is known to exacerbate the manifestations of lead exposure. Acute adult lead exposure leads to renal proximal tubular damage. Chronic exposure causes renal dysfunction characterized by hypertension, hyperuricemia, gout, and chronic renal failure. Once in the blood, lead is distributed primarily among three compartments — blood, soft tissue (kidney, bone marrow, liver, and brain), and mineralizing tissue (bones and teeth).

Other possible sources of lead
▶▶ Tobacco
▶▶ Crayons
▶▶ Lead crystal glasses
▶▶ Lead paint
▶▶ Lead pipes
▶▶ Newspapers and magazines containing lead-based ink
▶▶ Various cosmetics
▶▶ Hair colorings
▶▶ Toothpaste
▶▶ Water from old faucets or old pipes
▶▶ Bowls or dishes made by hand
▶▶ Cans
▶▶ Herbs from other countries

Cadmium

The largest sources of airborne cadmium in the environment are the burning of fossil fuels, such as coal or oil, and the incineration of municipal waste materials. Cadmium may also be emitted into the air from zinc, lead, or copper smelters.

Smoking is another important source of cadmium exposure. Smokers have about twice as much cadmium in their bodies as do non-smokers. Persons who smoke one or more packs of cigarettes per day show mean blood Cd concentrations (2 ug/l) tenfold over those of non-smokers (about 0.2 ug/l) — in range of blood concentrations causing bone loss in animals. Cadmium in cigarettes may be an important factor in osteoporosis in people who smoke; in non-smokers, food is generally the source of cadmium exposure. Cadmium levels in some foods can be increased by the application of phosphate fertilizers or sewage sludge to farm fields.

*Cadmium is highly toxic and is more toxic
than lead or mercury.*

Cadmium reduces the activity of 5'-deiodinase, which catalyzes conversion of thyroxine to reverse triiodothyronine (rT3) in peripheral tissues, which causes fatigue. It decreases the level of glutathione present in the liver and damages the liver. and causes cross-linking of the body's endogenous nucleic acids, proteins, and lipids and stimulates the production of free radicals.

Cadmium interferes with bone formation and causes osteomalacia and osteoporosis. It is strongly implicated as a cause of enlarged prostate (it stimulates the growth of the epithelium of the prostate) and increases the risk of prostate cancer (due to its antagonism of zinc and selenium cadmium, can replace zinc in the prostate).

Cadmium raises blood pressure via kidney damage and increases the incidence of calcium kidney stones.

Cadmium reduces the body's production of antibodies, IgG, and IgM, which increases susceptibility to bacterial and viral diseases. Try using wooden bowls and wooden utensils.

Rest and sleep

Go to bed by 10 pm, and get a minimum eight hours of sleep per night without interruptions. Sleep rejuvenates the mind and body while enhancing the natural cycle of healing and rest that takes place every night. Sleep helps to organize memories, solidify learning, and improve concentration. Proper sleep, especially sleep where you are actively dreaming (REM sleep), regulates mood as well. Sleep is cumulative; if you lose sleep one day, you feel it the next. If you miss adequate sleep several days in a row, you build up a "sleep deficit," which impairs the following:

➤ Motor skills
➤ Information processing
➤ Judgment
➤ Irritability and crankiness
➤ Reaction time
➤ Short-term memory
➤ Vision
➤ Increases driver fatigue

Sex two to three times per week

Practicing safe sex is of the utmost importance, however if you are in a stable relationship there are some real benefits to have sex on a regular basis.
These benefits include:
➤ Lowers mortality rates.
➤ Reduces risk of prostate cancer.
➤ Improves posture.
➤ Boosts self esteem.
➤ Makes a person feel younger.
➤ Firms tummy and buttocks.
➤ Keeps spouses connected emotionally.
➤ Offers pain-relief.
➤ Gives people a positive attitude on life.
➤ Reduces risk of heart disease.
➤ Makes a person calmer.
➤ Makes a person less irritable.
➤ Reduces depression.
➤ Allows for better bladder control.
➤ Relieves menstrual cramps.
➤ Helps people sleep better.
➤ Improves digestion.
➤ Improves memory.

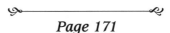

▸▸ Produces chemicals in the brain to stimulate the growth of new dendrites.

▸▸ Lowers the level of cortisol, a hormone that can trigger fatigue.

▸▸ Helps people achieve weight loss, since about 200 calories are burned during 30 minutes of active sex.

No liquid two hours before bed

Also avoid caffeine or stimulants at night. Remember the digestive track for liquids is faster than for solids, so it's logical to stop drinking liquids two to three hours before going to sleep.

No food four hours before bed

Your activity slows down at night and your metabolism drops. You are not burning energy as you do during the active part of the day and your body begins to store food as fat. So avoid eating before bedtime.

Exercise

The recommended routine would be to engage in some form of meditation (yoga, tai chi, Qi gan) an hour each day. One hour daily do some fast walking or 30 minutes of cardio vascular three times per week. Also important is 30 minutes of weight bearing exercise two times per week. Finally, be sure to practice deep breathing three times daily.

Clean environment

Use friendly biodegrading household cleaners and products free of formaldehyde. Use organic and natural hygiene products as well. It will be good for you and the environment.

Food additives

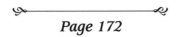

Food additives are substances intentionally added to food during manufacturing to increase the desirability of the finished food product. Additives can alter the color, texture, and stability of the food or reduce spoilage time. There are approximately 2000 different types of additives. The standard American diet includes three to five pounds of these additives per year. Additives can be toxic chemicals that can give rise to a number of symptoms. The most common are psychological or neurological, such as depression, headaches, mental fusion, mental illness, or abnormal nerve reflexes. Preservatives accumulate in body fat. The most common allergic reaction experienced is hives.

▸▸ Use products free of aspartame.

▸▸ Use products free of MSG (monosodium glutamate). It enhances the flavor of protein by exciting the taste buds. It can overexcite the nerve endings and cause symptoms known as "Chinese restaurant syndrome." Symptoms are reported as a burning sensation in the back of the neck, headaches, chest tightness, diarrhea, and flushing of the face.

▸▸ Use products free of hydrogenated or partially hydrogenated oil.

▸▸ Use products free of sodium or potassium (nitrate, nitrite, sulfite, sulphites, metabisulfite, and bisulfate) in any forms. Nitrite-nitrate toxicity is due to its affinity for the oxygen carrying molecule in the blood, hemoglobin. Nitrates convert hemoglobin to methemoglobin, which causes problems with oxygen transport. Heating nitrites, or their coming into contact with stomach acids, converts nitrites to nitromines, a substance known to cause stomach cancer. Nitrites and nitrates are added to meats to prevent the growth of bacteria that causes botulism. It also gives the classic pink color to processed meats. They are found in luncheon meats, ham, hot dogs, smoked fish, and baby foods.

▸▸ Salicylates are aspirin-like compounds used to increase or enhance the flavor of foods. Those allergic to aspirin can experience reactions from eating foods high in salicylates such as curry powder, paprika, thyme, dill, oregano, and turmeric. It is also found in the following prepared foods: cake mixes, pudding, ice cream, gum, soft drinks, and most dried fruits and berries. The average intake per day is 1 = 200 mg.

▶ Artificial dyes are widely used in foods, beverages, and drugs. The most common coloring agents used are called azo dyes (dyes impregnated with nitrate). Most are petroleum products derived from coal tar. Certain tissues in the body are more susceptible to dyes, especially those that have a quick turnover such as the cornea of the eye, tissue in the mouth, tissue lining the stomach and small intestine, and blood and lymph tissue. Use products free of any type of food coloring. Out of 33 known coloring agents, the following are the most commonly used.

Blue No. 2 -
Found in high amounts in cat food and soda pop.
It is implicated in causing brain cancer.
Citrus red - found in Florida oranges.
Green No. 3 - implicated in thyroid cancer.
Yellow No. 6 - Implicated in kidney cancer.
Yellow No.5 — Tartrazine (also known as "FD&C Yellow
Number 5" or "E-102" in Europe - is a coal-tar
derivative that is used to color foods, cosmetics, and other
products. It is literally industrial waste.

Tartrazine

Tartrazine is highly implicated in allergic responses and attention deficit disorder (ADD). Those allergic to aspirin might react to tartrazine. Tartrazine sensitivity is common in around 20 to 50% of individuals. It is a known inducer of asthma medications (aminophyline), and can be found in sedatives, steroids, antihistamines, and antibiotics. Vitamins can also contain tartrazine.

Tartrazine has been implicated in some cases of ADD, and consumption of tartrazine provokes the symptoms of ADD in some children. Tartrazine induces asthma in people who are susceptible to asthma. Tartrazine often causes hives. Tartrazine is not just a color; it is a complex product containing many different chemical compounds. It is used in drugs, especially shells of medicinal capsules, syrups, cosmetics, fruit cordial, colored fizzy drinks, instant puddings, cake mixes, custard powder, soups, sauces, ice cream, sweets, chewing gum, marzipan, jam, jelly, marmalade, mustard, yogurt, and many convenience foods together with glycerin, lemon, and honey products. It is also used with Brilliant Blue FCF to produce various green shades (i.e. for tinned processed peas).

Other foods containing tartrazine are:
- Orange drinks (Tang, Daybreak, Awake)
- Gelatin desserts (Royal and Jell-O)
- Italian dressing (Kraft)
- Cake mixes and icings (Pillsbury, Duncan Hines)
- Seasoning salt (French's)
- Macaroni and cheese (Kraft)

Other Chemical Names for tartrazine are 4,5-dihydro-5-oxo-1-(4-sulfophenyl)-4-[(4-sulfophenyl)azo]-1H-Pyrazole-3-carboxylic acid, trisodium salt, Dihydro-5-oxo-1-(4-sulfophenyl)-4-[(4-sulfophenyl)azo]-1h-pyrazole-3-carboxylic acid, trisodium salt, Pyrazole-3-carboxylic acid, 4,5-dihydro-5-oxo-1-(4-sulfophenyl)-4-[(4-sulfophenyl)azo]-, trisodium salt, Sulfophenyl-4-[(4-sulfophenyl)azo]-1h-pyrazole-3-carboxylic acid, trisodium salt,

Trisodium 1-(4-sulfophenyl)-4-[(4-sulfophenyl)azo]-1h-pyrazole-3-carboxylatec.

▸▸ Use products free of salicylates.
▸▸ Use products free of BHA (butylated hydroxyanisole). BHA is a synthetic antioxidant used as a preservative. High toxicity to liver.
▸▸ Use products free of BHT (butylated hydroxytoluene). BHT is commonly found in prepared and packaged foods such as breakfast cereals, chewing gum, and oil-containing products (i.e. potato chips, vegetable oils, and shortening). Causes toxicity and damage to lungs and liver.
▸▸ Use products free of calcium and potassium (benzoates). Benzoic acid and benzoates are widely used and are commonly found in shrimp and fish in extremely high amounts.
▸▸ Sulfites are typically used to prevent browning, color changes, or microbial spoilage. They are commonly sprayed on fresh fruit, vegetables, and fresh shrimp. The average person consumes 2-3 mg per day. If restaurants are the main source of meals, then an average of 150 mg per day is consumed. Sulfites destroy vitamin B1 and also cause asthma.
▸▸ Irradiation is a type of food additive that kills microorganisms and insects and inhibits sprouting of potatoes and onions. It also delays the ripening of fruit. The type of radiation used is called ionizing radiation, which produces URP's (Unique Radiolytic Products). Retail food must be labeled with this logo and the word "picowaved." The most common irradiated foods are spices, chicken, fruits, and vegetables.
▸▸ Sulfur dioxide destroys vitamin B1. Sulfur dioxide is absorbed via the blood and is excreted through the skin and lungs thereby contributing to body odor. Sulfur dioxide is a component of flatulence.

▸▸ Use products free of sugar and sugar substitutes.
▸▸ Avoid smoked foods, which contain benzpyrene — a proven cause of cancer.
▸▸ Avoid carbonated beverages.
▸▸ Avoid fast foods.
▸▸ Avoid deep fried food.
▸▸ Avoid food high in tyramine. The toxic effect of tyramine is often described as "the cheese effect," especially when tyramine-induced damage occurs as a result of the use of monoamine oxidase (MAO) inhibitors. Not all people are sensitive to tyramine — those who are sensitive to tyramine are susceptible to the following ailments:

1. Tyramine can increase blood pressure (increasing the risk of hypertension) by causing the release of catecholamines, especially in the presence of monoamine oxidase (MAO) inhibitor drugs.
2. People with high levels of candida albicans should avoid tyramine-containing foods.
3. Some people suffer from food allergies to tyramine-containing foods (due to tyramine causing the release of histamine from mast cells, which leads to the allergic reaction).
4. Tyramine can cause lethargy.
5. Tyramine causes over-stimulation of the adrenal glands (which results in depletion of the body's norepinephrine reserves).
6. Tyramine can cause anxiety (by over-stimulating the adrenal glands, which results in depletion of the body's norepinephrine reserves).
7. Tyramine can cause over-stimulation of the autonomic nervous system (ANS).
8. Tyramine can cause headaches.

Your Blood Tells All

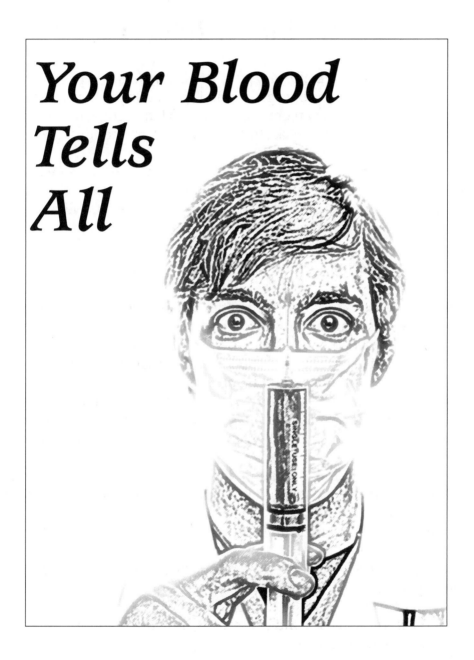

Your Blood Tells All

You need to realize you have a problem first

I always have my patients get a blood panel done before we start detox. It is like reading an encyclopedia of what is going on in their bodies. It also sets a baseline that we look at later to see what improvements have been made.

To the right in the sidebar is my own before and after. As I will tell you about in the Detox chapter (read more on page 90), I started eating as my patients do and then I detoxed. The results were extraordinary and very telling.

Blood work for males or females should be:
CBC

CBC is used as a broad screening test to check for such disorders as anemia, infection, and many other diseases. It is actually a panel of tests that examines different parts of the blood.

White blood cell (WBC) is a count of the actual number of white blood cells per volume of blood. There are five different types of white blood cells, each with its own function in protecting us from infection. The differential classifies a person's white blood cells into each type: neutrophils, lymphocytes, monocytes, eosinophils, and basophils.

Red blood cell (RBC) is a count of the actual number of red blood cells per volume of blood. Both increases and decreases can point to abnormal conditions.

Hemoglobin (Hgb) measures the amount of oxygen-carrying protein in the blood.

Hematocrit (HCT) measures the amount of space red blood cells take up in the blood. It is reported as a percentage.

Platelet count (PLT) is the number of platelets in a given volume of blood. Both increases and decreases can point to abnormal conditions of excess bleeding or clotting.

Mean platelet volume (MPV) is a machine-calculated measurement of the average size of your platelets. New platelets are larger, and an increased MPV occurs when increased numbers of platelets are being produced.

Mean corpuscular volume (MCV) is a measurement of the average size of your RBCs. When MCV is elevated when the RBCs are larger than normal (macrocytic), this is anemia caused by vitamin B12 deficiency. When MCV is decreased, RBCs are smaller than normal (microcytic); this is anemia of iron deficiency.

Mean corpuscular hemoglobin (MCH) is a calculation of the amount of oxygen-carrying hemoglobin inside the RBCs. Since macrocytic (B12 deficiency) RBCs are larger than either normal or microcytic (iron deficiency) RBCs, they tend to have higher MCH values.

Mean corpuscular hemoglobin concentration (MCHC) is a calculation of the concentration of hemoglobin inside the RBCs. Decreased MCHC values (hypochromia) are seen in conditions where the hemoglobin is abnormally diluted inside the red cells, such as in (iron deficiency) anemia and in thalassemia. Increased MCHC values (hyperchromia) are seen in conditions where the hemoglobin is abnormally concentrated inside the red cells, such as in hereditary spherocytosis, a relatively rare congenital disorder.

Red cell distribution width (RDW) is a calculation of the variation in the size of your RBCs.

Comprehensive metabolic panel

The comprehensive metabolic panel (CMP) is typically a group of 14 specific tests that are frequently ordered to give the doctor important information about the current status of your kidneys, liver, and electrolyte and acid/base balance, as well as of your blood sugar and blood proteins. The CMP is used as a broad screening tool to check organ function and check for conditions such as diabetes, liver disease, kidney disease, and hypertension. This test should be

Dr. Sokhandan
Blood Work results from
PACLAB Network Laboratories

**After 3 months of eating whatever
he wished, without consideration
for calories, fat content, and
toxins.**

Type	Result	Normal
Cholesterol	214	0-149
HDL	38L	40-59
LDL	151H	0-99
Glucose	89	65-114
DHEA-S04	370H	58-257
Vitamin D	27L	30-150
A1C	6.1	4.0-6.0
TSH	1.56	.40-5.00

After 4 weeks for detox.

Type	Result	Normal
Cholesterol	160	0-149
HDL	38L	40-59
LDL	105H	0-99
Glucose	69	65-114
DHEA-S04	307H	58-257
Vitamin D	54	30-150
A1C	5.5	4.0-6.0
TSH	1.56	.40-5.00

fasting, usually collected after a 10 to 12 hour fast (no food or liquids other than water).

Lipid panel

The lipid profile is used to guide providers in deciding how at-risk a person is for heart disease.

The lipid profile includes:
▸▸ Total cholesterol
▸▸ HDL (often called good cholesterol)
▸▸ LDL (often called bad cholesterol)
▸▸ Triglycerides
▸▸ VLDLs (very-low-density lipoproteins)
▸▸ Cholesterol/HDL ratio

LDLs and VLDLs are the so-called "bad" cholesterols. Unlike HDLs, LDLs and VLDLs are high-cholesterol particles. Cholesterol is necessary for various bodily functions. It is a precursor to all steroid hormones, including mineral-corticoids, glucocorticoids, and sex hormones, vitamin D, vital component of the myelin sheath and other important functions of cholesterol, athletic performance, regulating blood sugar, controlling blood pressure, regulating mineral balance, maintaining libido, and building muscle mass. However, too much cholesterol is harmful, since excess cholesterol can be deposited in blood vessel walls, and these fat deposits can lead to atherosclerosis (hardening of the arteries) and cardiovascular disease. Factors such as age, sex, and genetics influence our lipid profile. Certain aspects of our lifestyle, including diet, level of physical activity, level of blood sugar (diabetes control), and smoking, will affect our lipid profile. Some medical conditions can raise or lower cholesterol and triglyceride levels. People with personal or family history of CAD or peripheral vascular disease at an early age should test lipoprotein sub-fraction to assess their risk of developing heart disease. This helps monitor the effectiveness of lipid-lowering treatment and/or lifestyle changes, with the help of your doctor.

Thyroid hormone tests

A thyroid-stimulating hormone (TSH) blood test is used to check for thyroid gland problems. The thyroid gland makes hormones that regulate the way the body uses energy, and thyroid hormones are needed for normal development of the brain, especially during the first three years of life. The thyroid gland is a butterfly-shaped gland that lies in front of your windpipe (trachea), just below your voice box (larynx). The thyroid gland uses iodine from food to make two thyroid hormones, thyroxine (T4) and triiodothyronine (T3). The thyroid gland stores these thyroid hormones and releases them as they are needed. TSH is produced when the hypothalamus releases a substance called thyrotropin-releasing hormone (TRH). TRH then triggers the pituitary gland to release TSH.

Symptoms of an underactive thyroid are fatigue, feeling cold, weight gain, dry skin and hair, and constipation. In many cases, hypothyroidism runs in families. People who have relatives with thyroid disease should pay attention to symptoms and have occasional tests by their doctor. People with multiple sclerosis, type 1 diabetes, rheumatoid arthritis, and Addison's disease and other autoimmune disorders are at increased risk for hypothyroidism and should get tested regularly. Hypothyroidism is associated with increased rates of heart failure; people with congestive heart failure should be tested for thyroid problems. Menopausal women should also get their thyroid tested periodically.

Type of test — TSH, free T3, free T4

The free or unbound portion (free T4 or FT4, and free T3 or FT3 and rT3) more accurately represents what the body's true thyroid hormone levels are. Levels of free hormone represent the active hormone available to react with cell receptors in the body and TPO (detected auto antibodies directed against the enzyme thyroid peroxidase).

Vitamin B12 and folate

Vitamin B12 and folate are primarily ordered to help diagnose the cause of macrocytic anaemia. They can be requested as follow-up tests when large red cells and a decreased hemoglobin concentration are found during an RBC test. Folate and vitamin B12 may be used to help evaluate the nutritional status of a patient with signs of significant malnutrition or malabsorption. This may include those with alcoholism and those with disorders associated with malabsorption, such as celiac disease, Crohn's disease, and cystic fibrosis. Vitamin B12 and folate may also be ordered to help diagnose the cause of mental or behavioral changes, especially in young children and the elderly.

25(OH) vitamin D3

This blood test measures 25 hydroxy vitamin D and 1,25 dihydroxy vitamin D. 25 (OH) vitamin D is the major inactive form of the hormone found in the blood and is a precursor to the active hormone, 1,25 dihydroxy vitamin D. Because of its long half-life and higher concentration, 25 OH vitamin D is commonly measured to assess and monitor vitamin D status in individuals.

Vitamin D is the building block of a powerful steroid hormone in our body called calcitriol. Sunlight and vitamin D are critical to all life forms. The main function of vitamin D is to promote calcium, magnesium, iron, and zinc absorption in the gut and transfer across cell membranes, thus contributing to strong bones and teeth.

Vitamin D enhances the strength and efficiency of your immune system, which decreases your risk of developing autoimmune conditions like rheumatoid arthritis and lupus.

Vitamin D helps your body regulate its blood sugar levels, playing an important role in preventing type 2 diabetes.

Vitamin D helps to prevent high blood pressure.

Vitamin D will also enhance the uptake of toxic metals like lead, cadmium, aluminum, and strontium. Vitamin D supplementation should never be suggested unless calcium intake is sufficient or supplemented at the same time.

DHEA-sulfate

This test is used to evaluate the function of the adrenal gland. DHEA-sulfate is a weak androgen (male hormone) produced by the adrenal cortex in both men and women. The adrenal gland is one of the major sources of androgens in women (the other being the ovaries, which produce testosterone). The secretion and the blood levels of the adrenal steroid dehydroepiandrosterone (DHEA) and its sulfate ester (DHEAS) decrease profoundly with age. DHEA-sulfate is measured in women showing symptoms of virilism (male body characteristics) or hirsutism (excessive hair growth). It is also done in children who are maturing too early (precocious puberty).

Testosterone total and free

The level of testosterone rises during adulthood until it peaks around age 40, then it gradually decreases. Testosterone hormone is responsible for development of male secondary sexual characteristics. It is secreted by the adrenal gland and testes in men and by the adrenal gland and ovaries in women. A testosterone test can help to measure total and free, which provides a better understanding of how much testosterone is indeed available in the bloodstream. The concentration of free testosterone in the bloodstream is very low, typically < 2 % of the total testosterone concentration. The total testosterone consists of two forms of testosterone; one is bound to sex hormone binding globulin (SHBG), and the other is free-circulating testosterone unattached to serum proteins albumin. Testosterone levels can only be confirmed through lab testing. A test of total testosterone by serum (blood test) is usually sufficient, and urine or saliva testing will also work. People considering taking anti-aging medicines, such as human growth hormone (HGH) or steroids, should know their testosterone levels, which can be potentially dangerous to those drugs.

FSH (Follicle-stimulating hormone)
FSH is produced by the pituitary gland. As females approach menopause, FSH levels increase as estrogen levels decrease. The higher level FSH, the more likely females are to be in menopause. When a woman has not had her period for 12 months, clinically she is menopausal. FSH levels will fluctuate as estrogen levels fluctuate from month to month, and even from day to day. The FSH test may

also help women who have had a hysterectomy, but still have their ovaries. The FSH test is usually done to help diagnose problems with sexual development, irregular vaginal bleeding, infertility, menopause, ovarian cysts, and polycystic ovary disease.

LH (Luteininzing hormone)

Luteininzing hormone (LH) is a protein hormone released by the anterior pituitary gland. In women, an increase in LH levels at mid-cycle causes ovulation. In men, LH stimulates production of testosterone. An LH test is usually done to help diagnose anovulatory bleeding, infertility, menopause, polycystic ovary disease, and ovarian cysts.

PSA (Prostate-specific antigen)

Prostate-specific antigen is a protein produced by the prostate gland. Elevated PSA levels may indicate prostate cancer or a non-cancerous condition such as prostatitis or an enlarged prostate. A PSA level of 1.5 or higher indicates that you may have an enlarging prostate. A PSA test is used along with a digital rectal exam (DRE) to help detect prostate cancer in men age 50 and older. Some men (up to 30%) with prostate cancer have a normal PSA blood test, and up to 75% of men with a high PSA blood test do not have prostate cancer. Additionally, the PSA blood test cannot determine if the cancer is a slow-growing or aggressive cancer. It usually should follow with an ultrasound and prostate biopsy.

IGF-1 (Insulin-like growth factor - 1)

In adults, abnormally low levels of GH and/or IGF-1 may cause subtle, non-specific symptoms such as:
▸ Adverse lipid changes

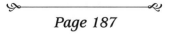

‣ Fatigue
‣ Decreased bone density
‣ Reduced exercise tolerance

This test identifies diseases and conditions caused by deficiencies and overproduction of growth hormone (GH), to evaluate pituitary function, and to monitor the effectiveness of GH treatment. The IGF-1 test is an indirect measure of the average amount of GH being produced by the body. IGF-1 and GH are peptide hormones, small proteins that are vital for normal bone and tissue growth and development. GH is produced by the pituitary and secreted into the bloodstream throughout the day and night, with peaks that occur mostly during the night. IGF-1 is produced, primarily in response to GH stimulation, by the liver, and some is also produced by skeletal muscles. It mediates many of the actions of GH and so stimulates the growth of bones and other tissues and promotes the production of lean muscle mass. IGF-1 mirrors GH excesses and deficiencies, but its level is stable throughout the day, making it a useful indicator of average GH levels.

SHBG (Sex hormone binding globulin)

The sex hormone binding globulin (SHBG) test measures the concentration of SHBG in the blood. SHBG is a protein that is produced by the liver. It binds tightly to estradiol, dihydrotestosterone (DHT), and testosterone and transports them in the blood in a metabolically inactive form. The amount of SHBG in circulation is affected by age and sex, by decreased or increased testosterone or estrogen production, and can be affected by certain diseases and conditions such as liver disease, hyperthyroidism or hypothyroidism, and obesity. Changes in SHBG concentrations can in turn affect the amount of testosterone that is available to be used by the body's tissues. Normally, about 40 to 60% of testosterone is bound to SHBG, and the rest is weakly and reversibly bound to albumin (protein). Only about 2% is immediately available to the tissues as free testosterone. Testosterone that is not bound (free) can also be checked if a man is having sexual problems for deficiency. In women, concern is excess testosterone production and symptoms such as amenorrhea, acne, hirsutism, infertility, and polycystic ovarian syndrome (POS).

Recommended for both men and women, other hormones such as estradiol, luteininzing hormone, and prolactin should be evaluated.

Homocysteine

Homocysteine is a toxic, endogenous sulphydryl — containing amino acid — a homologue of cysteine. A homocysteine test measures the amount of the amino acid homocysteine in the blood. High levels of homocysteine are closely associated with many forms of cardiovascular disease. Homocysteine facilitates the deposition of cholesterol around the heart. This buildup may increase the blood clots in the lungs (pulmonary embolism) or deep veins of the legs (deep venous thrombosis). Homocysteine is the underlying cause of osteoporosis, and elevated homocysteine contributes to the onset and progression of Alzheimer's disease. Twenty-five to 29% of vegetarians have elevated homocysteine due to low or lack of methionine and vitamin B12 in their diets.

Cardio CRP (C-reactive protein)

C-reactive protein is a test which measures the concentration in blood serum of a special type of protein produced in the liver and a type of endogenous protein that is present during episodes of acute inflammation or infection. In the body, CRP plays the important role of interacting with the complement system and immunologic defense mechanism. The complement system is a group of proteins (that work with the immune system) that move freely through the bloodstream. CRP is a biomarker of cardiovascular disease risk, atherosclerosis, Crohn's disease, fracture, inflammation, insulin resistance, pancreatitis, and rheumatoid arthritis.

Blood work for females over 35 should be:

- ▸▸ CBC
- ▸▸ Comprehensive metabolic panel
- ▸▸ Lipid panel
    Cholesterol
    Triglyceride
    HDL
    LDL
    VLDL
- ▸▸ TSH, free T3, free T4, and rT3
- ▸▸ 25(OH) vitamin D3
- ▸▸ DHEA sulfate
- ▸▸ Testosterone total and free
- ▸▸ Estradiol

Blood work for persons with risk factors

Blood work for those who have a risk of heart disease or who might be pre-diabetic suffering from some dizziness – or woman with a low total cholesterol count should have the following tests done:
- ▸▸ Cholesterol
- ▸▸ Triglyceride
- ▸▸ HDL
- ▸▸ LDL
- ▸▸ VLDL
- ▸▸ Lipoprotein sub-fraction
- ▸▸ VAP test

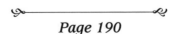

Have a clear picture of your problems and your symptoms. Generally, you only see your doctor when you are unwell to look at one particular aspect of your health which you are suffering from; do your research and seek a professional and ask as many questions as needed until you understand your symptoms or your problems. Stress has many symptoms, and common symptoms include anxiety, difficulty concentrating, depression, headache, sleep disorders, short-temper, and upset stomach. Some of those signs can be mistaken for other diseases if you are not familiar with your body or lack the knowledge regarding the problems.

Do not ignore the symptoms that caused discomfort.
Amenorrhea, or cessation of your menstrual cycle
Cold and flu symptoms
Digestive tract problems (constipation, diarrhea)
Disorientation or nausea
Depression or panic attacks
Excess sweating during sleep
Hot flashes, mood changes, vaginal dryness
Headaches which do not release with rest
Excess urination, thirst, and hunger
Enlarged lymph nodes
Irregular heartbeat with fatigue
Light-headedness
Localized bone pain
Lumps and bumps on the lower leg
Lung problems
Pressure in the chest
Unusual fatigue
Other symptoms you usually do not have

Avoid a quick fix

Always get a second opinion and ask as many questions as needed about the problem from your health care professional. Don't be worried about hurting someone's feelings. What you might be doing is hurting yourself by not insisting on receiving the most possible information about you condition so that you can make informed decisions.

Other factor detriments to health

- ▸▸ Low calories diets.
- ▸▸ Not enough rest.
- ▸▸ Heavy exercise.
- ▸▸ Chronic stress.
- ▸▸ Working too much.
- ▸▸ Working night shifts.
- ▸▸ Drinking alcohol more than three times a week.
- ▸▸ Not enough sunlight.
- ▸▸ Lack of fresh air.

How can you protect your body against the toxins?

- ▸▸ Recognize which organs need detox (digestive system, liver, kidney).
- ▸▸ Detox two times a year.
- ▸▸ Detox for a minimum of three weeks (digestive system, kidney, and liver).
- ▸▸ Use the right detox medicines.
- ▸▸ Use proper food combining (non-allergen food) during detox.
- ▸▸ Avoid over-the-counter herbal and supplements for detox and maintaining health.

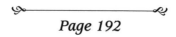

Conclusion

By understanding and utilizing the above factors, you will experience the greatest improvement in your health, and your perspective will shift from symptomatic relief to understanding and facilitating the body's potent, innate healing systems. You will notice a boost in your immune system, improved vitality, improved mobility, increased energy, improved sleep, weight control, balanced emotion, improved sexual desire, and improved cell integrity for a younger look.

For ordering detox medicines and instructions,
go to www.rebootyourbody21.com.

Blood types

Do you know what your blood type is? If not, you may want to ask your physician to order a special blood test for you to determine what your blood type is. There has been extensive scientific research over the past 30 years that shows evidence that your individual blood type determines your predisposition toward getting certain diseases such as cancer, heart disease, diabetes, lupus, muscular sclerosis, allergies, etc. Your blood type also determines what type of biochemistry your digestive system is made of. "Your blood type is a powerful genetic fingerprint that identifies you as surely as your DNA."

There are four blood type groups: O, A, B, and AB. The letter in the blood type refers to the type of antigen that is in the blood, so blood type 'A' has the 'A' antigen and so on. Blood type O is the only type that has no antigens and therefore those with type O blood become universal donors. Blood types are also identified as positive or negative. Those with positive blood types contain the RHD antigen, People with negative blood must receive blood types that are also negative, however people with the RHD positive can receive either positive or negative. Here is what the various types mean in relation to your health.

Blood type O

Blood type O is the oldest blood type; it evolved around 40,000 BC. This is the blood type associated with carnivores, because the stomach produces a high level of hydrochloric acid, which is necessary to digest protein. Blood type O people have the hardiest digestive systems and they are carnivores (meat-eaters). People with blood type O digest protein (animal) much easier and they need it for good health, as well as vegetables and fruits. Carbohydrates and dairy products should be kept to a minimum; they cannot digest carbohydrates or dairy very well, especially wheat products containing gluten.

Blood type O should avoid drinking coffee, since coffee will increase production of stomach acid even more, and this tends to make them prone to ulcers (peptic), especially if they are constantly under a great deal of stress. Green tea should be substituted for coffee for their caffeine craving.

Blood type O people have a tendency to have low thyroid, low metabolism, and depression.

Exercises for blood type O
‣ Fast walking or jogging
‣ Weight training

Foods that should be avoided, which cause weight gain
‣ Brussels sprouts, corn, cabbage,

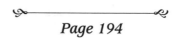

▶ cauliflower, kelp, kidney beans, lentils,
▶ mustard greens, navy beans, wheat, and sugar.
▶ Foods which encourage weight loss
▶ Seafood: bluefish, cod, hake, halibut, herring, mackerel, pike, rainbow trout, red snapper, salmon, sardines, shad, snapper, sole, striped bass, sturgeon, swordfish, tilefish, white perch, whitefish, yellow perch, yellowtail, and sea kelp (for iodine)
▶ Red meat: beef, buffalo, lamb, veal, and venison
▶ Vegetables: broccoli, kale, and spinach

Other foods that should be avoided
▶ Pork: bacon and ham
▶ Seafoods: catfish, caviar, herring (pickled), and smoked salmon
▶ Dairy products: all varieties of cheeses, milk, whey, and yogurt
▶ Oils: corn oil, cottonseed oil, peanut oil, and safflower oil
▶ Nuts & seeds: Brazil nuts, cashews, peanuts,
▶ Pistachios, and poppy seeds
▶ Grains & pastas: bulgur wheat flour, couscous, flour, durum wheat flour, semolina pasta, spinach, pasta, sprouted wheat flour, white flour, whole wheat flour.
▶ Vegetables: avocado, cauliflower, white & yellow corn, eggplant, shiitake mushrooms, olives (black, Greek, Spanish), potatoes (red & white), and alfalfa sprouts
▶ Fruits: blackberries, coconuts, melon (cantaloupe & honeydew), oranges, plantains, rhubarb, strawberries, tangerines
▶ Spices: capers, cinnamon, cornstarch, corn syrup, nutmeg, black & white pepper, vinegar (apple cider, balsamic, red & white wine)

Blood type A

This blood type evolved between 25,000 and 15,000 BC. People

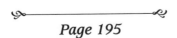

with blood type A have weak digestive systems. Blood type A cannot tolerate or digest animal protein or dairy well and are usually lactose intolerant. They should be vegetarian due to lack of or insufficient hydrochloric acid in their stomach. Blood type A should consume fruits, legumes, tofu, whole grains, and vegetables. Blood type A people do not absorb vitamin B12 properly from the foods they eat. Vitamin B12 is normally found in red meat, therefore supplementing the diet with vitamin B12 is critical (sublingually). Other supplementation, like digestive enzymes and betaine, is recommended.

Exercises for blood type A
‣ Tai chi
‣ Yoga
‣ Golfing
‣ No heavy or vigorous workouts

Foods that cause weight gain
‣ Dairy products, kidney beans, lima
‣ beans, meat, sugar, and white
‣ flour

Foods that help with weight loss
‣ Vegetables, olive oils, flaxseed and flaxseed oil, pineapple, and soy products

Other foods to avoid
‣ All meats: beef, buffalo, duck, goose, lamb, pheasant, pork, poultry, rabbit, veal, venison, and quail
‣ Seafood: anchovy, barracuda, bluefish, catfish, caviar, all shellfish (clam, crab, lobster, oysters, scallop, shrimp) crayfish, eel, flounder, frog, gray sole, haddock, hake, halibut, herring (fresh & pickled), mussels, octopus, sole, squid (calamari),

smoked salmon, striped bass, and tilefish
- ▶▶ Oils: corn oil, cottonseed oil, peanut oil, safflower oil, and sesame oil
- ▶▶ Nuts & seeds: Brazil, cashews, and pistachios
- ▶▶ Beans & legumes: garbanzo, kidney, lima, navy, and red beans
- ▶▶ Breads & grains: English muffins, high-protein bread, matzos, wheat, multi-grain bread, pumpernickel, semolina, wheat bran muffins, whole wheat bread
- ▶▶ Fruits: bananas, coconuts, mangoes, melon (cantaloupe, honeydew), oranges, papayas, rhubarb, and tangerines
- ▶▶ Spices: capers, plain gelatin, pepper (black, cayenne, peppercorns, red pepper flakes, white), vinegar (apple cider, balsamic, red and white wine)
- ▶▶ Beverages: beer, distilled liquor, seltzer water, all sodas, black teas

Blood type B

Blood type B developed between 15,000 and 10,000 BC. Persons with blood type B have great (tolerant) digestive systems which can tolerate most foods, with a few exceptions that should be avoided (corn, buckwheat, lentils, peanuts, and sesame seeds). Blood type B should avoid gluten from wheat and wheat germ, which can cause hypoglycemia (low blood sugar). Blood type B have much less of a problem digesting dairy products. Blood type B should avoid chicken.

Food that increases weight:
- ▶▶ Dairy products

Foods that encourage weight loss
- ▶▶ Green vegetables, lamb, rabbit, turkey, pheasant, eggs, low-fat dairy products, seafood from deep ocean fish (cod, flounder,

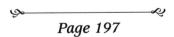

The doctor as patient

Whenever I talk to my patients and tell them what they need to do to improve their health and well being, not only now but many years into the future, they look at me and say — "sure it is easy for you, you don't have health issues, or weight issues." They see my trim body shape and don't realize what I go through everyday to maintain my weight and my health. I am just as human as my patients, desiring foods that are no good for me. However I know that if I eat sweets I will crave sweets.

I recommend that everyone watch the movie "Super Size Me," a documentary which asks the question "why is America so fat." Director Morgan Spurlock ate all of his meals at McDonalds for a period of 30 days. The results for his health and weight were both startling and downright scary. This documentary and the comments from my patients about my lack of understanding inspired me to

(Continued next page, boxed column)

halibut, salmon, and sole), licorice tea (great to sip after a meal as this will prevent hypoglycemia), soy products, olive oil and flaxseed oil, oatmeal, oat bran, millet, rice bran, and spelt

Other foods to avoid
▸ Black-eyed peas, garbanzo beans, wheat, shellfish, tomatoes, tofu, artichokes, avocados, olives (black, green, Greek, and Spanish), pumpkin radishes, and mung bean
▸ Oils: canola oil, corn oil, cottonseed oil, peanut oil, safflower oil, sesame oil, sunflower oil, and coconut oil
▸ Fruits: persimmons, pomegranates, pears, rhubarb, and star fruit
▸ Spices: black and white pepper, and cinnamon
▸ Condiments: almond

extract, barley malt, corn syrup, ketchup, plain gelatin, tapioca
▶ Beverages: hard distilled liquor, seltzer water, and all sodas

Blood type AB

Very rare, and the gentle offspring of type A and type B blood, this blood type has only been around for about 1000 years; a modern adaptation and result of intermingling of disparate groups. Less than 5% of the world's population have blood type AB. You combine the best and the worst of blood types A and B. Most foods that are bad for the type A and type B person are also bad for the type AB person, with the exception of tomatoes. The blood type AB person can tolerate tomato lectins well. Like type A, they do not produce enough hydrochloric stomach acid to digest animal protein well, such as red meat and

personal experiment of my own. I started by having my blood work done while I was on my regular routine for optimum health. Then I began eating like my patients do — consuming mindlessly whatever is set in front of me at the table. I became a creature of habit, thinking about my daily activities, problems, whatever was happening around me, but never about me. I gave no time or thought about my own health or what I was putting in my mouth.

I have to confess, I never went to McDonalds for a Big Mac and fries, nor did I drink a lot of soda. But I did start to make all my favorite pastries. Whenever I was hungry I ate, including snacking after dinner which I never do normally. I did this for 2-1/2 months.

Interestingly, during this time, I noticed that I was turning to food for comfort. I wasn't feeling as well as I normally do. And although my regular routine is to graze all day long on walnuts, almonds or fruit, when I started having a regular lunch I found

(Continued next page, boxed column)

I was very tired afterwards. A big lunch also meant I would be hungry a couple of hours later. Once established I knew that overcoming food cravings was going to be difficult.

After indulging my every hunger whim and taste bud fantasy for 10 weeks I found that I had gained 11 pounds. When I stopped I knew it would take my body 3 times as long, 30 weeks, to recover from what took me 10 weeks to create.

Now I had to detox, and the trouble was I had uncontrollable cravings, I was on an emotional roller coaster, my concentration was poor, and my energy was depleted. Even my sleep was interrupted. I really craved sugar and my body wanted it to boost my energy.

I detoxed and then I redid my blood work. My vitamin D decreased to the lowest it had ever been. Further my blood work would have been received by most general practitioners as a reason to prescribe medication for diabetes and high cholesterol.

(Continued next page, boxed column)

poultry, yet they do need some animal protein. Therefore, portion size is important, and with less frequency. Be sure to take bromelain, a digestive enzyme derived from pineapple, to assist with the digestion of animal protein meals. The best meats for type AB are lamb, mutton, rabbit, and turkey. Also, avoid smoked and cured meats.

Foods that encourage weight gain
▸▸ Red meat, kidney beans, lima beans, seeds, corn, buckwheat, and wheat
▸▸ Foods that encourage weight loss
▸▸ Tofu, seafood, dairy, green vegetables, spirulina, sea kelp, and pineapple

Other foods to avoid
▸▸ Meat: bacon, beef, ground beef, buffalo, chicken, Cornish hen,

duck, goose, ham,
partridge, pork, veal,
venison, and quail
▶▶ Seafood: anchovies,
barracuda, beluga,
bass (bluegill, sea,
striped), shellfish
(clams, conch, crab,
lobster, oysters,
shrimp), flounder,
frog, haddock, halibut,
herring (pickled),
smoked salmon,
octopus, sole, bass,
turtle, and yellowtail
▶▶ Cheese: all kinds
▶▶ Oils: corn oil,
cottonseed oil,
safflower oil, sesame
oil, and sunflower oil
▶▶ Nuts & seeds: poppy
seeds, pumpkin
seeds, sesame butter
(tahini), sesame seeds,
sunflower butter, and
sunflower seeds
▶▶ Legumes: black beans,
fava beans, garbanzo
beans, kidney beans,
lima beans (dry),
mung beans, and
black-eyed peas
▶▶ Grains & pasta:

If I had started taking drugs for cholesterol, sooner or later I would have heart problems. If I had starting taking a drug for diabetes I could have had complications with my digestive system or my thyroid gland. Either way I would have been doomed with obesity.

How did I stay on track, once I went back to detox and a regimen for optimum health. First I had to sit myself down and concentrate on getting into the right frame of mind. What is more important health or a slice of white bread. I also knew that I could take supplements that would suppress my now eager appetite to ease the way. For sugar cravings I ate more fruit, or drank a glass of water before I ate. I wrote down what I was eating, because keeping a journal of food intake helps me in facing my responsibility to myself. I also wrote what I was feeling emotionally when I was craving food and tried to analyze what was really going on. Would eating really solve the problem or

(Continued next page, boxed column)

make me feel better? The answer is always no.

I know it is difficult to lose weight or change lifelong habits. I have a recent patient that has lost 67 pounds in 5 months. Every time she finds herself craving foods she shouldn't eat I change the detox plan (I have 5 distinct plans that I utilize in my practice). The change is always crafted to renew her commitment and resolve her cravings. She has become quite good now at handling her own cravings and she is now on a new automatic pilot.

I learned from this experience. I became even more compassionate about what my patients go through. I understand the dilemma and the difficulty with sticking to a health program — after all they are addicted to food just as I had become during my experiment.

SEE APPENDIX A on page 274 for my before and after blood work and explanation of the damage done by changing my diet.

buckwheat kasha, barley flour, and soba (buckwheat) noodles
▶▶ Vegetables: artichoke (domestic & Jerusalem), avocado, corn (white & yellow), lima beans, black olives, peppers (green, jalapeno, red, yellow), and radishes
▶▶ Fruits: bananas, coconuts, guava, mangoes, oranges and orange juice, persimmons, pomegranates, prickly pears, rhubarb, and star fruit

For more information about your blood type read Dr. Peter J. D-Adamo (*Eat Right for Your Type*).

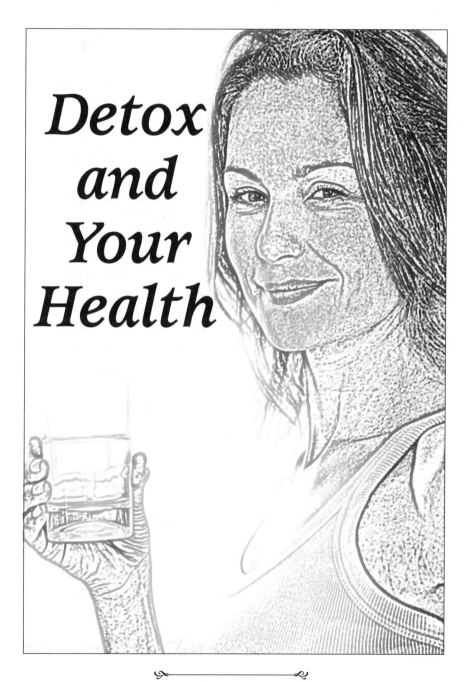

Detox
and
Your
Health

Detox and your health

Now that you have learned what you need to do to improve your eating and your lifestyle, the next step is to detox. Detoxing cleanses the body of toxins naturally and is the first step to changing bad habits to good ones. Any chemicals that your body has become dependent on will be removed from your system during this process.

It is time to service your engine, just like you periodically change the oil in your car. Or think of how you brush and floss twice daily, yet you still go to the dentist for a deep cleaning twice a year.

Your body is no different. To detox is a preventive precaution to rid the body of all the garbage you have digested and inhaled. Even if you already eat healthy you can't avoid all the toxins, and these toxins accumulate over time. Detoxing will help to clean the colon, liver, lymphatic system, gall bladder pancreas, lungs, and skin. It is important to know that no matter your age or how healthy you think you are you do need to detox.

Think about how good it feels when you have your teeth cleaned at the dentist. You can't help but rub your tongue over the surface of your teeth. This is what you will feel inside, clean. Gone will be fatigue, bloating, weight gain, insomnia, and so on.

Now take a few minutes to answer the questionnaire and see if now is the right time to take this all-important next step.

When do we know it is time for a detox?

Do you feel tired, lethargic, or sluggish?
    No   Rarely   Often
Do you have difficulty concentrating or have slow or fuzzy thinking?
    No   Rarely   Often

Do you feel depressed or have mood swings?
No   Rarely   Often
Do you get more than one or two colds per year?
No   Rarely   Often
Do you get post-nasal drip, congestion, or "stuffed up" in your nose or sinuses?
No   Rarely   Often
Do you have bad breath, a coated tongue, a bitter or metallic taste in your mouth?
No   Rarely   Often
Do you have body odor?
No   Rarely   Often
Do you have strong-smelling urine?
No   Rarely   Often
Do you have trouble sleeping or feel unrested upon waking?
No   Rarely   Often
Do you have sore muscles or joints?
No   Rarely   Often
Do you have weak or brittle nails?
No   Rarely   Often
Do you have dark circles under your eyes?
No   Rarely   Often
Do you have digestive disturbances such as bloating, gas, or indigestion a couple of hours after eating?
No   Rarely   Often
Do you have less than one bowel movement per day?
No   Rarely   Often
Do you feel anxious or stressed out?
No   Rarely   Often
Do you have sensitivity to odors, foods, or chemicals
No   Rarely   Often
Do you have allergies?
No   Rarely   Often

Do you have eczema, dry skin, acne, or skin rashes?
   No   Rarely   Often
Do you gain weight easily?
   No   Rarely   Often
Do you have food cravings?
   No   Rarely   Often
Do you have pain or discomfort under your right rib cage?
   No   Rarely   Often
Does dietary fiber cause constipation?
   No   Rarely   Often
Do you feel like you're not as healthy as other people your age?
   No   Rarely   Often

These are all potential signs of the need for general detoxification. Evaluate the function of cellular mechanisms and eliminative mechanisms, including urinary, liver, and bowel function.

For detoxing, you need to follow step-by-step directions and always consult with your physician first.

Health assessment questionnaire

Based on your responses to the health assessment questionnaire, you will be able to access the type of detoxification program necessary for your optimum health. Always consult with your physician first.

✔ Check any of the items below that you consume on a daily basis:

Diet

☐ Dairy ☐ Coffee ☐ Caffeinated tea ☐ Carbonated beverages

☐ Candy or other sweets ☐ Artificial sweeteners ☐ Margarine

- [ ] Alcohol [ ] Luncheon meats/hot dogs [ ] Fried food
- [ ] Red meat [ ] Farm-raised fish [ ] Shellfish [ ] Canned goods
- [ ] Refined flour/baked goods [ ] Fast food [ ] Chewing tobacco
- [ ] Cigars/pipes [ ] Cigarettes [ ] Water, tap [ ] Water, filtered
- [ ] Water, well [ ] Diet often [ ] Vitamins/minerals
- [ ] Organic food

Medications

Check any medications you're currently taking or have taken in the last three months:

- [ ] Antacids [ ] Antibiotics [ ] Antidepressants [ ] Antifungals
- [ ] Anticonvulsants [ ] Aspirin [ ] Ibuprofen [ ] Asthma inhalers
- [ ] Beta blockers [ ] Chemotherapy [ ] Cortisone
- [ ] Diabetic medications [ ] Diuretics [ ] Hormone therapy
- [ ] Estrogen/progesterone [ ] Heart medication
- [ ] High blood pressure medication [ ] Laxatives
- [ ] Insulin [ ] Oral/implant contraceptives [ ] Radiation exposure
- [ ] Recreational drugs [ ] Relaxants/sleeping

☐ Thyroid medication

☐ Tylenol/acetaminophen ☐ Ulcer medication

Other medications and dosages (if known)

_____

Now look at each section and check if you have any of these symptoms. (For more information on the suggested supplements you may want to visit www.rebootyourbody21.com)

Section 1

☐ Stomach upset with vitamins ☐ Feel better if you do not eat

☐ Diarrhea or loose stool ☐ Bad heartburn or acid reflux

☐ Stomach pain ☐ Belching or gas within half-hour of meal

☐ Loss of taste for meat ☐ Bloating after meal

☐ Skip breakfast ☐ Sleepy after meal ☐ Sweat has a strong odor

☐ Fingernails chip, peel, or break easily

☐ Vegan (no meats, fish, dairy, or eggs)

☐ Sense of fullness after meals ☐ Anemia unresponsive to iron

☐ Undigested food in stools ☐ Dark or tarry stools

If you have any three or more of the above symptoms you can use the suggested supplements. Always consult with your physician first.

Suggested supplements
Batine plus
Digestive Enzyme
Vitamin C
L-glutamine
Multi-vitamin (men's, women's with or without iron)
EPA/DHA

Section 2

☐ Chronic fatigue or fibromyalgia ☐ Gallbladder attacks

☐ Stomach upset with greasy food ☐ Gallbladder removed

☐ Pain between shoulder blades ☐ Bitter taste in mouth after meals

☐ Greasy or shiny stool ☐ Pain under right side of rib cage

☐ Headache over the eyes ☐ Nausea ☐ Dry or itchy skin

☐ Itchy feet or skin peels on feet ☐ Light or clay-colored stool

If you have any three or more of the above symptoms you can click to suggested supplements. Always consult with your physician first.

Suggested supplements
Vitamin C
L- glutamine
L- phenylalanine
MSM
Gluco-ton
Multi-vitamin
EPA/DHA

Section 3

☐ History of hepatitis ☐ Long term use of prescription medication

☐ Exposure to diesel fumes ☐ Sensitive to tobacco smoke

☐ Sensitive to chemicals
(perfume, cleaning solvents, insecticides, exhaust, etc.)

☐ Bothered by food additives (aspartame, MSG, etc.)

☐ Hemorrhoids or varicose veins ☐ History of morning sickness

☐ Motion (car, sea, or airplane) sickness

☐ Hangover after drinking alcohol ☐ Recovering alcoholic

☐ Getting sick after consuming alcohol

If you have any three or more of the above symptoms you can click to suggested supplements. Always consult with your physician first.

Suggested supplements
L- carnitine
L- cysteine
L- glutamine
Detox
EDTA
Cholesterol formula
Vitamin C
EPA/DHA
Multi-vitamin

Section 4

☐ Food allergies ☐ Sensitivity to wheat ☐ Airborne allergies

☐ Sensitivity to dairy ☐ Sinus congested, "stuffy head"

☐ Asthma ☐ Experience hives or skin rashes ☐ Crohn's disease

☐ Crave carbohydrates ☐ Abdominal bloating after meals

☐ Alternating constipation and diarrhea

If you have any three or more of the above symptoms you can click to suggested supplements. Always consult with your physician first.

Suggested supplements
L- glutamine
Probiotic
Querce-plex
Vitamin C
MSM
Digestive enzyme
Batine plus

Section 5

☐ Crave carbohydrates Coated tongue ☐ Crave carbohydrates

☐ Crave carbohydrates ☐ Stool hard or difficult to pass

☐ History of yeast infection ☐ Stools are flat or ribbon shaped

☐ Dark circles under eyes ☐ Stools are not well formed (loose)

☐ Nail fungus, ring worm, athlete's foot

☐ Excessive foul-smelling lower bowel

☐ Anus itching ☐ Bad breath or strong body odors

☐ History of parasites ☐ Cramping in lower abdominal region

☐ Less than one bowel movement per day ☐ Mucus in stool

If you have any three or more of the above symptoms you can click to suggested supplements. Always consult with your physician first.

Suggested supplements
Batine plus
Digestive enzyme
L-arginine
L-glutamine
MSM
Querce-plex

Section 6

☐ History of fractures ☐ Shorter than you used to be

☐ Bone loss (reduced density on bone scan) ☐ Morning stiffness

☐ Joint pop and click ☐ History of herniated disc

☐ Pain or swelling in joints ☐ History of bone spurs

☐ Bursitis or tendonitis ☐ History of carpal tunnel syndrome

If you have any three or more of the above symptoms you can click to suggested supplements. Always consult with your physician first.

Suggested supplements
Osteo support
Glucosamine/MSM
Multi-vitamin
EPA/DHA
Vitamin D3
Vitamin C

Section 7

☐ Calf, foot, or toe cramp at rest ☐ Gag easily

☐ Cold sores, fever blisters, or herpes lesions

☐ White spots on fingernails ☐ Crave chocolate

☐ Cuts heal slowly ☐ Tendency to anemia

☐ Scar easily ☐ Difficulty swallowing

☐ Decreased sense of taste or smell

☐ Lump in throat ☐ Hoarseness ☐ Dry mouth, eyes, or nose

☐ Small bump on side of your arms

If you have any three or more of the above symptoms you can click to suggested supplements. Always consult with your physician first.

Suggested supplements
Multi-vitamin
EPA/DHA
Vitamin D3
Vitamin C
Detox
EDTA
L-arginine
DIM

Section 8

☐ Crave fatty or greasy food ☐ Afternoon headache

☐ Tension headaches ☐ Low fat diet (past or present)

☐ Dry flaky skin and/or dandruff

☐ Headaches when out in the sun ☐ Muscles easily fatigued

If you have any three or more of the above symptoms you can click to suggested supplements. Always consult with your physician first.

Suggested supplements
Detox
EDTA
Vitamin C
Vitamin D3
Multi-vitamin
EPA/DHA
Vitamin B12 drop
Ubiquinol (Coenzyme Q10)

Section 9

☐ Crave sweets ☐ Sleepy in afternoon ☐ Eat sugary snacks

☐ Hard to fall sleep ☐ Binge or uncontrolled snacks

☐ Frequent thirst ☐ Crave coffee or sweets in afternoon

☐ Frequent urination ☐ Fatigue that is relieved by eating

☐ History of diabetes in family ☐ Irritable before meals

☐ Excessive appetite ☐ Shaky if meal is delayed

☐ Headache if meals are skipped or delayed

☐ Awaken a few hours after falling sleep

If you have any three or more of the above symptoms you can click to suggested supplements. Always consult with your physician first.

Suggested supplements
Gluco-tone
Vitamin C
Vitamin D3
EPA/DHA
Detox
EDTA
L-carnitine
Ubiquinol (Coenzyme Q10)
Querce-plex

Section 10

☐ Feel worse or sore after exercise ☐ Heart races

☐ Wake up without remembering dreams ☐ Night sweats

☐ Muscles become easily fatigued ☐ Loss of muscle tone

☐ Bleeding gums when brushing teeth

☐ Ringing in the ears/tinnitus ☐ Strong light at night irritates eyes

☐ Restless leg syndrome ☐ Small bumps on back of arms

☐ Cheilosis (cracks in corner of mouth) ☐ Polyps or warts

☐ Vulnerable to insect bites ☐ Fragile skin ☐ MSG sensitivity

If you have any three or more of the above symptoms you can click to suggested supplements. Always consult with your physician first.

Suggested supplements
L-carnitine
L-arginine
Ubiquinol (Coenzyme Q10)
Cholesterol formula
Vitamin C
EPA/DHA
Multi-vitamin

Section 11

☐ Difficulty falling sleep ☐ Salt foods before tasting

☐ Slow starter in the morning ☐ Afternoon yawning

☐ Tend to be a "night person" ☐ Afternoon headache

☐ Hyper and trouble calming down ☐ Chronic fatigue

☐ Jittery with caffeinated drink

☐ Pain on the medial or inner side of knee

☐ Clench or grind teeth ☐ Allergies and/or hives

☐ Headache after exercise ☐ Asthma ☐ Crave salty food

If you have any three or more of the above symptoms you can click to suggested supplements. Always consult with your physician first.

Suggested supplements
L-tyrosine
L-phenylalnine
7-keto
Gluco-tone
Vitamin C
EPA/DHA
Multi-vitamin

Section 12

☐ Difficulty losing weight ☐ Loss of lateral one-third of eyebrow

☐ Nervous, difficulty working under pressure ☐ Seasonal sadness

☐ Fast pulse at rest ☐ Morning headache wears off during day

☐ Flush easily ☐ Chronic constipation ☐ Sensitive to cold

☐ Intolerance to high temperatures ☐ Mentally sluggish

☐ Poor circulation (cold hands and/or feet)

☐ Easily fatigued, sleepy during day ☐ After long sleep still tired

☐ Excessive hair loss and/or coarse hair

   If you have any three or more of the above symptoms you can click to suggested supplements. Always consult with your physician first.

Suggested supplements
L-tyrosine
L-phenylalnine
L-arginine
Sleep formula
Vitamin C
Vitamin D3
EPA/DHA
Multi-vitamin
Gluco-ton

Section 13

☐ Urination difficult or dribbling ☐ Decreased sexual function

☐ Prostate problems ☐ Interruption of stream during urination

☐ Difficult to start and stop urine stream

☐ Pain on inside of legs or heels ☐ Pain or burning with urination

☐ Feeling of incomplete bowel evacuation

☐ Waking up to urinate at night

If you have any three or more of the above symptoms you can click to suggested supplements. Always consult with your physician first.

Suggested supplements
Prostate Health
7-keto
Vitamin D3
Selenium
Ubiquinol (Coenzyme Q10)
EPA/DHA
Multi-vitamin
Vitamin C

Section 14

☐ Mood swings associated with periods (PMS)

☐ Crave chocolate around periods ☐ Depression during periods

☐ Excessive menstrual flow ☐ Scanty blood flow during periods

☐ Vaginal discharge ☐ Breast fibroids, benign masses

☐ Endometriosis ☐ Uterine fibroids

If you have any three or more of the above symptoms you can click to suggested supplements. Always consult with your physician first.

Suggested supplements
EPA/DHA
Vitamin D3
Probiotic
Sleep formula
7-keto
L-tyrosine
Ultra indinal
Vitamin C
Multi-vitamin

Section 15

☐ Occasional skipped periods ☐ Variations in menstrual cycles

☐ Painful intercourse (dyspareunia) ☐ Vaginal dryness

☐ Vaginal itchiness ☐ Excess facial or body hair

☐ Gain weight around hips, thighs, and buttocks

☐ Hot flashes ☐ Night sweats (in menopausal females)

☐ Thinning skin

If you have any three or more of the above symptoms you can

click to suggested supplements. Always consult with your physician first.

Suggested supplements
Ultra indinal
Vitamin D3
7-keto
Black cohash
Glucoton
EPA/DHA
Vitamin C
Multi-vitamin

Section 16

☐ Runny or dripping nose ☐ Itchy skin/dermatitis

☐ Frequent cold or flu ☐ Cysts, boils, or rashes

☐ Catch cold at beginning of winter ☐ History of Epstein bar virus

☐ History of herpes ☐ History of chronic fatigue ☐ Acne (adult)

☐ Frequent infection (ear, sinus, lung, bladder, skin, etc.)

☐ History of immune suppuration ☐ History of chronic fatigue

☐ History of urinary infection ☐ History upper respiratory infection

If you have any three or more of the above symptoms you can click to suggested supplements. Always consult with your physician first.

Suggested supplements
Vitamin D3
Vitamin C
Ubiquinol (Coenzyme Q10)
Qurceplex
Selenium
EPA/DHA

The stages of detox

Stage one of detox

In the first stage of detox we need to prepare the body and give the support for detoxification. As we know, many people over age 25 have gone through many yo-yo diets for weight loss. Another component for detox is a weak immune system — when we get sick all the time, or at least three times per year, get flu shots during winter time, or have allergies. Gastrointestinal problems are another factor which I pay attention to. If your digestion is compromised, no matter what you consume will pass through without absorption. In this stage we need to support all the organs with the right nutrients, supplementation, and exercise.

In this stage you will take:
1- Multi-vitamin for your gender — three capsules two times/day with meals
2- Opti EPA (fish oil) — two capsules two times/day with meals
3- Vitamin C — two capsules two times/day away from the meals
4- L-glutamine — two capsules three times/day with meals
5- Synerpan-5 — two capsules two times/day with meals
6- Glucoton — two capsules three times/day with meals

7- Probiotic — two capsules one time/day with meal

Before you start this program, you should consult with your physician if you have any health concerns. In this stage, which takes four weeks, you should not consume any caffeine, dairy, alcohol, wheat, or sugar. In this stage you should also avoid foods that you have an allergic reaction to. In this stage you may experience some symptoms of withdrawal such as body aches, headache, nausea, and fatigue.

You should drink six to eight glasses of water per day. At the end of this stage, you may lose some weight, and some of your symptoms that you had before might clear up (headache, allergy, insomnia, etc.)

Stage two of detox

In this stage you should consume six to eight glasses of water/day and follow with these supplements.

1- Detox — two capsules three times/day with meals

2- EDTA — two capsules three times/day with meals

3- Vitamin C — two capsules two times/day between meals

4- Opti EPA — two capsules two times/day with meals

5- Multi-vitamin — two capsules three times/day with meals

6- Glucoton — two capsules three times/day with meals

7- Cholesterol formula — two capsules three times/day with meals

In this stage your blood sugar and cholesterol, if they were in the high range, may become in the normal range. Also in this stage of detox, you may lose up to 10 pounds of your body weight. It is highly suggested to do blood work before and after your detox, and you have to remember that this may be an extra cost for you since your insurance will not cover your second test.

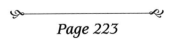

In this stage you will follow the:

DETOXIFICATION DIET II / Allergy Elimination
Prepared by Dr. Said Sokhandan ND, LAC
(modified from Tracking Down Hidden Food Allergies by William Crook, M.D.)

Purpose: To help free the body from some of the toxins that have accumulated in your system and identify hidden food allergens that may be causing some or all of your symptoms and health problems. During the detox and elimination period, all common allergens are completely eliminated from the diet and help the body detox for three weeks. After your symptoms improve, foods are added back, one at a time, to determine which foods provoke symptoms.

FOODS YOU MUST AVOID
DAIRY PRODUCTS — Milk, cheese, butter, yogurt, sour cream, cottage cheese, whey, casein, ice-cream, sodium caseinate, calcium caseinate, or any food containing these.

SOY PRODUCTS — If you have any allergic reaction.

WHEAT — Most breads, spaghetti, noodles, pasta, most flour, baked goods, durum semolina, farina, and man gravies, etc.

CITRUS FRUITS — Oranges, grapefruits, lemons, limes, tangerines/satsumas, and foods containing citrus. Also NO bananas, cantaloupe, honeydew, strawberry, or grapes.

COFFEES, TEAS, ALCOHOL — Must avoid caffeinated and decaffeinated coffee, as well as standard (such as Lipton) tea and decaffeinated tea. Herb teas are OK, except those containing citrus.

REFINED SUGARS — Including table sugar and any foods that contain it: candy, soda, pies, cake, cookies, etc. Other names for sugar include: sucrose, glucose, dextrose, corn syrup, corn sweetener, fructose, maltose, and laevulose. These must all be avoided. Some patients will be allowed 1-3 teaspoons per day of pure, unprocessed honey, maple syrup, or barley malt. This will be decided on an individual basis. Those restricted from all sugars should not eat dried fruit. Others may eat unsulphured (organically grown) dried fruits sparingly.

ORGANIC HONEY, MAPLE, OR BARLEY SYRUP — Not allowed.

FOOD ADDITIVES — Including artificial colors, flavors, preservatives, texturing agents, artificial sweeteners, etc. Most diet sodas and other dietetic foods contain artificial ingredients and must be avoided. Grapes, prunes, and raisins that are not organically grown contain sulfites and must be avoided.

ANY OTHER FOOD YOU EAT MORE THAN THREE TIMES A WEEK — Any food you are now eating three times a week or more should be avoided and tested later.

KNOWN ALLERGENS — Avoid any foods you know you are allergic to, even if it is allowed on this diet.

TAP WATER — Drinking (includes cooking) — Not allowed. If tap water is not allowed, use spring or distilled water bottled in glass or heavy plastic. Water bottled in soft (collapsible) plastic containers tends to leach plastic into the water. Some water filtration systems do not take out all potential allergens. Take your water with you, including to work or restaurants.

READ LABELS! Hidden allergens are frequently found in packaged foods. "Flour" usually means wheat, "vegetable oil" may mean corn oil, and casein and whey are dairy products. Make sure your vitamins are free of wheat, corn, sugar, citrus, yeast, and artificial colorings. Vary your diet, choosing a wide variety of foods. Do not rely on just a few foods, as you may become allergic to foods you eat every day.

FOODS YOU MAY EAT: (Preferably ORGANIC)

CEREALS (HOT) — Oatmeal, oat bran, cream of rye, Rice and Shine. (DRY) — Puffed rice, puffed millet, Oatio's (wheat-free), Good

Shepherd (wheat-free), Crispy Brown Rice Cereal. Diluted apple juice with apple slices, including all berries (no strawberry) and nuts go well on cereal. May use soy milk that has no corn oil added (such as some Eden Soy products; please read the ingredients carefully). Also may use almond nut milk. Most of these foods are available in health food stores or your supermarket.

GRAINS AND FLOUR PRODUCTS — 100% brown rice cakes, brown rice crackers, rye crackers; any 100% rye or spelt bread with no wheat; Oriental noodles, such as 100% buckwheat soba noodles; soy, rice, potato, buckwheat, and bean flours; rice or millet bread (as long as they do not contain dairy, eggs, sugar, or wheat); cooked whole grains including oats, millet, barley, buckwheat groats (kasha), rice macaroni, spelt (flour and pasta), brown rice, wild rice, amaranth, and quinoa. Most of these grains are available at health food stores.

LEGUMES (BEANS) — Includes soybeans, tofu, lentils, peas, chickpeas, navy beans, kidney beans, black beans, string beans, and others. Dried beans should be soaked overnight at least 12 hours. Pour off the water and rinse before cooking and no salt added during your cooking. Canned beans often contain added sugar or other potential allergens. Some cooked beans packaged in glass jars can be used as long as they contain no sugar.

Read labels. May also use bean dips without sugar, lemon, or additives. Canned soups including split pea and lentil soup (without additives) are OK. Soak all beans for 24 hours before cooking to release all gases within the lids of the beans.

VEGETABLES — Use a wide variety. All vegetables EXCEPT CORN.

Cooked vegetables: Allowed   Steamed: Allowed   Raw: Allowed

PROTEINS — Poultry and fowl allowed, fresh fish allowed, but no farm-raised fish (such as tuna and salmon, packed in spring water). Shrimp and most canned or packaged shellfish (such as lobster, crab, and oysters) may contain sulfites and should be avoided. Canned tuna, salmon, and other canned fish are OK.

Lamb rarely causes allergic reactions and may be used even when other meats are restricted. Also recommended are grain/bean casseroles (recipes in vegetarian cookbooks).

- Free-range/organic poultry: Allowed
- Free-range/organic red meats: Not allowed
- Lamb: Allowed
- Pork: Not allowed
- Shellfish: Not allowed
- Wild fish: Allowed
- Eggs: Not allowed

NUTS AND SEEDS — Nuts and seeds, either raw or roasted, without salt or sugar. To prevent rancidity, nuts and seeds should be kept in an airtight container in the refrigerator. May also use nut butters from health food stores or your supermarket, or from fresh ground nuts. Almond butter, cashew butter, and nut butter go well on celery sticks and crackers.

- Almonds/almond butter: Allowed
- Peanuts/peanut butter: Not allowed
- Cashews/cashew butter: Not allowed
- Walnuts/walnut butter: Not allowed
- Sesame/sesame butter: Not allowed

OILS AND FATS — Use cold-pressed or expeller-pressed oils (available from health food stores or your supermarket), as they are safer for the heart and blood vessels. Do not use corn oil or "vegetable oil" from an unspecified source, as this is usually corn oil.

Absolutely NO margarine or partially hydrogenated oil.

- Extra virgin olive oil (on SALADS ONLY): Allowed

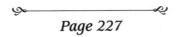

➤ Grape seed oil (cooking ONLY): Allowed
➤ Extra virgin coconut oil (cooking ONLY): Allowed
➤ Canola oil: Not Allowed
➤ Flaxseed (edible linseed) oil: Not allowed
➤ Sunflower oil: Not allowed
➤ Safflower oil: Not allowed
➤ Sesame oil: Not allowed
➤ Peanut oil: Not allowed
➤ Soy oil: Not allowed

SNACKS — Any food can be eaten as a snack, any time of day. Also suggested are celery, carrot sticks, or other vegetables; fruit in moderation (no citrus); and unsalted fresh nuts (almonds).

BEVERAGES — Herb teas (no lemon or orange), spring water, or filtered water in glass bottles.

THICKENERS — Rice, oat, millet, barley, soy, or amaranth flours; arrowroot, agar.

SPICES AND CONDIMENTS — Salt in moderation, pepper, turmeric, herbal spices (without preservatives, citrus, or sugar), garlic, ginger, onions, organic catsup and mustard (without sugar), wheat-free tamari sauce, Bragg liquid aminos, and vitamin C crystals in water, as a substitute for lemon juice.

MISCELLANEOUS — Sugar-free spaghetti sauce, fruit jellies without sugar or citrus, soups such as split pea, lentil, turkey/ vegetable, etc.

RECOMMENDED — Attach a filter to your shower head, which will help eliminate the amount of inorganic chlorine, which is a compound that is present in tap water, which then is disposed in your shower. Fifty to 80% of the inorganic chlorine that is present in a hot shower vaporizes into a toxic compound of chloroform, which is an odorless gas that is inhaled during the shower process. The amount of toxins absorbed through inhalation and through the pores in your skin from one shower is equivalent to drinking six to eight glasses of tap water.

SUGGESTION — Blood work should be done before you start the detox and also at the end of your 21 days, before introducing the foods which have been eliminated during detox. Results of your blood should show how your system is working and what suggestions should be taken by your physician.

1- CBC
2- Comprehensive metabolic panel
3- Lipid profile including VLDL
4- TSH, T4 total, T3 total
5- Homocysteine
6- CRP

GENERAL SUGGESTIONS
DO NOT RESTRICT YOUR CALORIES!

Start with a good breakfast, eat frequently throughout the day, and consume at least six to eight glasses of water (filtered) per day. If you do not eat enough, you may experience symptoms of low blood sugar, such as fatigue, irritability, headache, and too-rapid weight loss. To ensure adequate fiber, eat beans, permitted whole grains, whole fruits and vegetables, homemade vegetable soup, nuts, and seeds. Be sure to chew thoroughly, about 15-20 times, in order to enhance digestion.

PLAN YOUR MEALS FOR THE WEEK. TAKE A LIST WITH YOU to your supermarket or health store. If your schedule is very busy and it is hard to think of what to fix, take some time before starting the detox to make a list of all of your favorite types of foods and possible meal plans. For ideas, look through cookbooks that specialize in hypoallergenic diets, or recipes at the end of this book. Most meals can be modified easily to meet the requirements of the detox, without changing the meal plan for the rest of your family.

When you go to the supermarket or health food store, ask for assistance in locating "allowed" versions of breads, crackers, cereals, puffins, soups, etc.

Some people find it helpful to prepare additional foods on the weekend to cut down on thinking and preparation time during the week. If you need further assistance or ideas for meal preparation, go to the recipe section.

DINING OUT

Do not hesitate to ask questions or make requests. For instance, you could ask for fish topped with slivered almonds, cooked without added seasoning, butter, or lemon. Get baked potato with a slice of onion and tomato on top. Order grilled chicken or lamb chops with fresh vegetables, also prepared without added seasonings (with the exception of garlic and plain herbs). Use salad bars that do not use sulfites as a preservative and bring your own dressing (oil and cider vinegar with chopped nuts/seeds and fresh herbs). Get into the habit of carrying pure water, snacks, seasonings, etc., wherever you go to supplement your meals or to have something on hand if you start to get hungry.

WITHDRAWAL SYMPTOMS

About one in four patients develop mild "withdrawal" symptoms within a few days after starting the diet. Withdrawal symptoms may include fatigue, irritability, headaches, malaise, or increased hunger. These symptoms generally disappear within two to five days and are usually followed by an improvement in your original symptoms. If withdrawal symptoms are too uncomfortable, take buffered vitamin C, up to 1000mg, three times a day for several days. These products may be obtained from the office or from the Web site. In most cases, withdrawal symptoms are not severe and do not require treatment. It is best to discontinue all of the foods abruptly ("cold turkey"), rather than easing into the diet slowly.

TESTING INDIVIDUAL FOODS

It may take three weeks for symptoms to improve enough to allow you to retest foods. However, you may begin retesting after two weeks if you are sure you are feeling better. If you have been on the diet for four weeks and feel no better, contact the office for further instructions. Most patients do improve. Some feel so well on the diet that they decide not to test the foods — this could be a mistake. If you wait too long to retest, your allergies may "settle down" and you will not be able to provoke your symptoms by food testing. Then, you will not know which foods you are allergic to. If reintroducing certain foods causes a recurrence of symptoms, you are probably allergic to those foods. Food sources for testing should be pure sources of a food. For example, do not use pizza to test cheese, because pizza also contains wheat and corn oil. Do not use bread to test wheat, as it contains other ingredients.

Organic sources are the best to use for testing, as you will not experience interference from pesticides, hormones, or other additives, which may be used in commercial preparations. Test one new food each day. If your main symptom is arthritic pain, test one new food every other day. Allergic reactions to tested foods usually occur within 10 minutes to 12 hours after ingestion. However, joint pains may be delayed by as much as 48 hours. Eat a relatively large amount of each test food. For instance, on the day to test milk, add a large glass at breakfast, along with any of the other foods on the "permitted" list. If after one serving your original symptoms come back, or if you develop a headache, bloating, nausea, dizziness, or fatigue, do not eat that food anymore and place it on your "allergic" list. If no symptoms occur, eat the food again for lunch and supper and watch for reactions. Even if the food is well tolerated, do not add it back into your diet until you have finished testing all of the foods. If you do experience a reaction, wait until your symptoms have improved before testing the next food.

If you wake up the next morning with head or joint pain, nausea, or any other suspicious symptom, you may be experiencing a delayed reaction to the food you tested the day before. If you are uncertain whether you have reacted to a particular food, remove it from your diet and retest it four to five days later. You do not have to test foods you never eat.

Do not test foods you already know cause symptoms.

Foods may be tested in any order. Begin testing on a day you are feeling well (without colds, unusual headaches, flu, or body ache). Review the list of symptoms to watch for and keep a journal of how you feel.

Dairy test — Test milk and cheese on separate days. You may wish to test several cheeses on different days, since some people are allergic to one cheese but not another. It is usually not necessary to test yogurt, cottage cheese, or butter separately.

Wheat test — Use Wheatena (with no milk or sugar) or another pure wheat cereal. May add soy or nut milk.

Citrus test — Test oranges, grapefruits, lemons, and limes. Test these individually on four separate days. The lemon and lime can be squeezed into water. In the case of orange and grapefruit, use the whole fruit.

Fruit test — Try banana, grapes, cantaloupe, honeydew, and strawberry individually on five separate days.

Frequently eaten foods — Test tap water, if you have eliminated it, followed by those foods you have restricted (such as foods being consumed more than three times a week).

Optional tests — The following foods and beverages are considered undesirable, regardless of whether or not you are allergic to them. If any of them are not now a part of your diet, or if you are fully committed to eliminating them from your diet, there is no need to test them. However, if you have been consuming any of them regularly, it is a good idea to test them and find out how they affect you. Reactions to these foods and beverages may be severe in some cases. They should be tested only on days that you can afford to feel bad.

Coffee and tea tests (separate days) — Do not add milk, non-dairy creamer, or sugar. May add soy milk. If you use decaffeinated coffee, test it separately. Coffee, tea, decaffeinated coffee, and decaffeinated tea are separate tests.

Sugar test — Put 4 teaspoons of sugar in a drink or on cereal, or mix with another food. Try to skip this test if you can, the majority of people have allergies to sugar.

Chocolate test — Use 1-2 tablespoons of pure baker's chocolate or Hershey's cocoa powder.

Alcohol test (test this last) — Beer, wine, and hard liquor may require testing on different days, as the reactions to each may be different. Have two drinks per test day, but only if you can afford not to feel well that day and possibly the next day.

Calories

Your total daily calorie intake should be determined by your weight and energy expenditure. You should not lose more than one to two pounds per week. If you lose more than one or two pounds per week, you will start to lose muscle mass and slow your basal metabolic rate (BMR), which makes it harder to continue your weight loss. To lose one pound of fat per week, you have to burn 3500 calories. You need to burn 500 calories per day or decrease 500 calories per day. Remember, the key to weight loss is to lose weight primarily from fat. You should always eat a good diet.

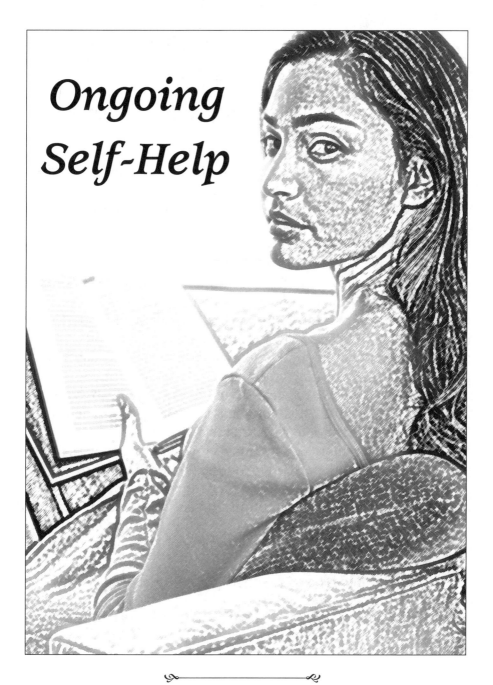

Ongoing Self-Help

Suggestions for Ongoing Self-Help

IF YOU ARE ALLERGIC TO ANY FOODS

Rotation diets — If you have an allergic constitution and eat the same foods every day, you may eventually become allergic to them. After you have discovered which foods you can eat safely, make an attempt to rotate your diet. A four-day schedule is necessary for some severely allergic patients, but most people can tolerate foods more frequently than every four days. You may eventually be able to tolerate allergenic foods, after you have avoided them for six to12 months. However, if you continue to eat these foods more frequently than every fourth day, the allergy may return.

Use common sense and consume a wide variety of foods. Do not just latch onto a few favorites. If you are rotating foods, be sure to avoid all forms of the food when you are on an "off" day. For instance, if you are rotating corn, be sure to avoid corn chips, corn oil, corn sweeteners, etc., except on the days that you are eating corn and corn products. It is not necessary to do strict food rotation during the elimination and retesting periods.

Watch for other allergic reactions — if you have an allergic constitution, you may be allergic to foods other than those you have eliminated and tested on this diet. Pay attention to what you are eating, and if you develop symptoms, review your recent meals and try to identify what may be different in what you have eaten. You can then eliminate that food for two weeks and test it again to see if you can provoke the same symptoms.

Try to eat organic food as much as possible, especially leafy vegetable, fruits, legumes, and proteins.

Eat small meals all day; this helps control your weight.

SYMPTOMS THAT MAY BE DUE TO FOOD ALLERGY

▸ General: Fatigue, anxiety, depression, insomnia, food cravings, obesity.

▸ Infections: Recurrent colds, urinary tract infections, sore throats, ear infections, yeast infections.

▸ Ear, nose, and throat: Chronic nasal congestion, postnasal drip, fluid in the ears, Meniere's syndrome.

▸ Gastrointestinal: Irritable bowel syndrome, constipation, diarrhea, abdominal cramping, ulcerative colitis, Crohn's disease, gallbladder disease.

▸ Lipids: Increased cholesterol, increased LDL.

▸ Cardiovascular: High blood pressure, arrhythmia, angina.

▸ Dermatologic: Acne, eczema, psoriasis, canker sores (aphthous ulcers), hives.

▸ Rheumatologic: Muscle aches, osteoarthritis, rheumatoid arthritis.

▸ Neurologic: Migraines and other headaches, numbness.

▸ Miscellaneous: Asthma, frequent urination, teeth grinding, bed-wetting, infantile colic.

Note: Most of these disorders have more than one cause, but food allergy is a relatively common and frequently overlooked cause.

Stage three of detox

A simple fasting plan will help dump more toxins out of the body.

You need to consult with your physician if you have any health issues. Be responsible for your health; this is only a suggestion and the responsibility is in your hands. During your detox stage three you need to take these supplements:

1- Detox — two capsules three times/day with meals

2- EDTA — two capsules three times/day with meals

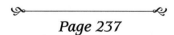

3- Vitamin C — two capsules two times/day away from the meals

4- Qurceplex — two capsules three times/day with meals

▸▸ **Day one:** organic fruits (all varieties except banana), cantaloupe, grapes, strawberry, and all citrus fruits.

▸▸ **Day two:** organic vegetable broth only (all varieties of vegetable), no corn.

▸▸ **Day three:** water only (if you have any health concerns, you should not do this stage and you should always consult with your physician first). Day three you can substitute with vegetables instead of water.

▸▸ **Day four:** repeat the vegetable broth as on day two.

▸▸ **Day five:** back to fruits as on day one.

▸▸ **Day six:** go back to your diet in stage two detox for seven days. If you lost 5% of your total weight from stage one, then you should do blood work and compare with your lab results from before; if you still have some unresolved issues, go to stage four.

Stage four of detox

In this stage you become vegetarian for four weeks and take these supplements:

1- Detox — two capsules three times/day with meals

2- EDTA — two capsules three times/day with meals

3- Vitamin C — two capsules two times/day between meals

4- Opti EPA — two capsules two times/day with meals

5- Multi-vitamin — two capsules three times/day with meals

6- L-glutamine — two capsules three times/day with meals

7- Vitamin B12 (sublingual) — 10 drops once/day between meals

After this stage you should have a greater understanding about your body and your health. Do not forget to have fun in your life and remember food is just one component of your health. This is my belief: let your food be your medicine and your medicine be your food.

Conclusion

By understanding the detox and utilizing the above factors, you will experience the greatest improvement in your health, and your perspective will shift from symptomatic relief to understanding and facilitating the body's potent, innate healing systems. You will notice a boost in your immune system, improved vitality, improve mobility, increased energy, improved sleep, weight control, balanced emotion, improved sexual desire, and improved cell integrity for a younger look.

Substances
that Help
to Detox

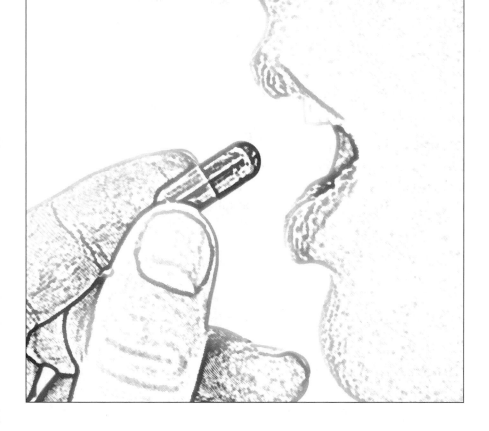

Substances that help to detox

N-acetyl-cysteine (NAC)

N-acetyl-cysteine is an endogenous pre-acetylized form of amino acid cysteine produced from cysteine within the body. N-acetyl-cysteine is a natural sulfur-containing amino acid derivative containing nutrients which play several critical roles in the body, including detoxification and protecting cells and cellular components against oxidative stress. NAC readily crosses cell membranes, even in HIV-infected cells. NAC is more stable than cysteine and is also more water soluble and therefore more bioavailable than cysteine. It is a very powerful antioxidant and free radical scavenger and helps protect the body from a variety of harmful agents.

- NAC prevents the destruction of glutathione (by preventing the oxidation of glutathione).
- NAC enhances the activity of glutathione-S-transferase.
- NAC facilitates the excretion of arsenic, mercury (chelate) Mercury from the body.
- Cases exist where humans affected by chronic arsenic poisoning have been saved from death when administered NAC upon arrival at the hospital.
- NAC deactivates the free radicals generated by hydrogen peroxide.
- NAC reduces the toxic effects of alcohol (ethanol) by functioning as a precursor for the endogenous production of glutathione.
- NAC helps to prevent alcohol-induced liver damage and fatty liver.
- NAC reduces the inflammation associated with colitis.
- NAC is an effective treatment for kidney stones (where kidney stones are caused by calcium oxalate or cystine accumulation).

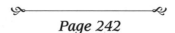

➤ NAC protects the body's endogenous protease inhibitor protein (alpha-1 antitrypsin) by preventing the oxidation of methionine residues within this protein.

➤ NAC helps to prevent the metastasis of many types of cancer.

➤ NAC enhances the ability of interleukin 2 (IL-2) to counteract cancer.

➤ NAC enhances the effectiveness of interferon alpha in the treatment of hepatitis C (primarily by counteracting the depletion of glutathione).

➤ NAC improves the function of white blood cells.

➤ NAC enhances the activity of NK lymphocytes.

➤ NAC (administered via aerosol spray inhaled) alleviates the symptoms of cystic fibrosis.

➤ NAC helps to prevent (diabetic) neuropathy in diabetes mellitus patients.

➤ NAC helps to prevent the free radical-induced destruction of beta cells in the pancreas of diabetes mellitus type 2 patients.

➤ NAC counteracts the excessive generation of free radicals in people who exercise.

➤ NAC prevents the exercise-induced destruction of glutathione (by preventing the oxidation of glutathione).

➤ NAC inhibits the replication of the hepatitis B virus that causes hepatitis B.

➤ NAC inhibits the oxidation of LDL cholesterol.

➤ NAC facilitates the detoxification function of the liver.

➤ NAC helps to prevent alcohol-induced liver damage.

➤ NAC helps to prevent alcohol-induced fatty liver.

➤ NAC improves some aspects of cognitive performance in Alzheimer's disease patients.

➤ NAC helps to prevent (diabetic) neuropathy.

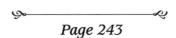

Alpha lipoic acid (ALA)

Lipoic acid, also known as lipoic acid (alpha lipoic acid) or thioctic acid, is a sulfurous compound that is considered sufficiently "essential" to be worthy of classification as a vitamin of the "B" group in modern orthomolecular circles — lipoic acid would have been classified as a vitamin except for the fact that it can be synthesized within the human body. It is a very important cofactor in the Krebs cycle (citric acid cycle), the body's main process for converting carbohydrates into energy. ALA is a medium length (eight carbon atoms) fatty acid containing two sulfur atoms. It is readily synthesized in the body and is well absorbed from the diet through the stomach and intestines.

- Lipoic acid inhibits damage to mitochondrial DNA (mtDNA) — the principal detrimental process implicit in the Mitochondrial DNA Theory of Aging.
- Lipoic acid helps to prevent atherosclerosis.
- Lipoic acid lowers blood pressure in hypertension patients.
- Lipoic acid helps to prevent age-related macular degeneration (ARMD) due to the antioxidant properties of lipoic acid; it can penetrate eye tissue and protect both the lens and the retina from degeneration.
- Lipoic acid reduces the risk of cataracts in diabetes mellitus patients and in normal, healthy persons.
- Lipoic acid inhibits the activation of aldose reductase (an enzyme that is implicated in cataracts due to its ability to catalyze the production of galacticol and sorbitol from galactose and glucose).
- Lipoic acid alleviates glaucoma.
- Lipoic acid is useful for the treatment of hepatitis C (especially when it is combined with selenium and milk thistle).
- Lipoic acid possesses antioxidant properties. (It functions as both a water-soluble and a fat-soluble antioxidant.)

➤ Lipoic acid increases the body's basal metabolic rate (BMR).

➤ Lipoic acid normalizes blood sugar levels.

➤ Lipoic acid increases energy levels in some chronic fatigue syndrome (CFS) patients.

➤ Lipoic acid prevents and alleviates many of the detrimental side effects that occur as a result of diabetes mellitus (both type 1 and type 2).

➤ Lipoic acid inhibits the ability of mercury to damage neurons.

➤ Lipoic acid acts as a coenzyme in the metabolism of carbohydrates.

➤ Lipoic acid improves the body's utilization of glucose within the muscles. ➤ Lipoic acid facilitates the conversion of glycogen into glucose.

➤ Lipoic acid protects superoxide dismutase (SOD) from oxidation.

➤ Lipoic acid improves the actions of insulin (mimics the function of insulin).

Lipoic acid increases intracellular glutathione levels by 30 to 70%.

➤ Lipoic acid inhibits the cross-linking (glycosylation) of some types of endogenous proteins (including albumin).

➤ Lipoic acid regenerates coenzyme Q10.

➤ Lipoic acid inhibits the excitotoxic effects of glutamic acid.

➤ Lipoic acid helps to protect the body from arsenic poisoning.

➤ Lipoic acid chelates (binds to and removes) accumulated cadmium from the body and helps to prevent cadmium from damaging the liver.

➤ Lipoic acid chelates (binds to and removes) accumulated mercury from the body.

➤ Lipoic acid inhibits the ability of mercury to damage neurons.

➤ Lipoic acid reduces the accumulation of lactic acid.

Ethylene diamine tetra acetic acid (EDTA)

EDTA removes toxic metals from the blood. Studies have shown that as people age they continuously accumulate toxic metals: lead, mercury, aluminum, iron, cadmium, and arsenic, among others. The accrual of these toxins invites an increased risk for various diseases, especially heart disease. The less of these metals we have in our bodies, the more likely we are to be physiologically healthy or simply feel good, and the lower our risk for heart disease. Because EDTA is so effective at removing unwanted metals and other minerals from the blood, it has been the standard, FDA-approved treatment for lead, mercury, aluminum, and cadmium poisoning for more than 50 years. EDTA normalizes the distribution of most metallic elements in the body.

EDTA helps prevent heart attacks, stroke, varicose veins, and more by inhibiting blood clotting. Because EDTA inhibits blood clotting so well, by tying up calcium, it is routinely added to blood samples that are drawn for testing purposes. Blood can't clot if the calcium is tied up. Inhibition of blood clotting can help prevent stroke, heart attack, phlebitis (painful inflammation of a vein), pulmonary embolism (potentially fatal clot to the lung), or varicose veins. Generally, these conditions are associated with aging.

EDTA makes stronger bones and reduces cholesterol by improving calcium and cholesterol metabolism. EDTA can help to lower cholesterol, the principal component of atherosclerotic plaque. Use of EDTA AND PROCAIN as an IV drip or push has great health benefits for athrosclorosis and heavy metal toxicity; you should consult your physician.

Health benefits of EDTA (used as a component of chelation therapy)
  ▸ EDTA improves the condition of the cardiovascular system. (Degeneration of the cardiovascular system is a major factor in the aging process.)

▸▸ EDTA helps to reverse cross-linking. (Cross-linking is an important factor in the progression of the aging process.)

▸▸ EDTA reverses calcification of the body's tissues. (The body's tissues become increasingly calcified with the progression of the aging process.)

▸▸ EDTA often terminates ventricular tachycardia.

▸▸ EDTA improves the flexibility of the walls (endothelium) of the arteries.

▸▸ EDTA helps to prevent the deposition of calcium and cholesterol in the atherosclerotic plaques that occur during the progression of atherosclerosis.

▸▸ EDTA improves blood circulation.

▸▸ EDTA alleviates age-related macular degeneration (ARMD).

▸▸ EDTA lowers total serum cholesterol levels.

▸▸ EDTA increases HDL cholesterol levels and lowers elevated LDL.

▸▸ EDTA can reverse many cases of gangrene (diabetic gangrene and atherosclerosis-induced gangrene).

▸▸ EDTA alleviates some cases of Alzheimer's disease. EDTA alleviates cerebral insufficiency. (By improving the function of blood vessels throughout the body, EDTA increases blood circulation to the brain.)

▸▸ EDTA improves memory in persons afflicted with memory impairment caused by cerebral insufficiency.

▸▸ EDTA helps to prevent (and possibly reverse) the calcification of the pineal gland.

Vitamin C

Vitamin C is required for the synthesis of collagen, an important structural component of blood vessels, tendons, ligaments, and bone. Vitamin C also plays an important role in the synthesis of the neurotransmitter, norepinephrine. Neurotransmitters are critical to brain function and are known to affect mood. In addition, vitamin C is required for the synthesis of carnitine, a small molecule that is essential for the transport of fat to cellular organelles called mitochondria, for conversion to energy. Recent research also suggests that vitamin C is involved in the metabolism of cholesterol to bile acids, which may have implications for blood cholesterol levels and the incidence of gallstones. Vitamin C is also a highly effective antioxidant. Even in small amounts vitamin C can protect indispensable molecules in the body, such as proteins, lipids (fats), carbohydrates, and nucleic acids (DNA and RNA) from damage by free radicals and reactive oxygen species that can be generated during normal metabolism, as well as through exposure to toxins and pollutants (smoking).

- ▸▸ Vitamin C protects the liver from the toxic effects of exposure to carbon tetrachloride.
- ▸▸ Vitamin C helps to detoxify several types of pesticides and inhibits the ability of pesticides to damage cells.
- ▸▸ Vitamin C inhibits the activity of aldose reductase.
- ▸▸ Vitamin C inhibits the activity of HMG-CoA reductase.
- ▸▸ Vitamin C inhibits the conversion of nitrites and nitrates to (carcinogenic) nitrosamines within the stomach.
- ▸▸ Vitamin C helps to lower elevated lipoprotein (a) levels.
- ▸▸ Vitamin C inhibits the production of prostaglandin E2 (PGE2).
- ▸▸ Vitamin C facilitates the excretion of arsenic from the body.
- ▸▸ Vitamin C facilitates the removal of cadmium from body and can reverse cadmium toxicity symptoms.
- ▸▸ Vitamin C inhibits the ability of cadmium to reduce the activity of 5'-deiodinase (the enzyme that catalyzes the conversion of thyroxine to triiodothyronine).
- ▸▸ Vitamin C facilitates the excretion of lead from the body.
- ▸▸ Vitamin C (1,000 mg per day) significantly reduces blood lead levels in tobacco smokers.
- ▸▸ Vitamin C lowers elevated blood histamine levels, and people who exhibit elevated blood histamine levels are often found to be deficient in vitamin C.

▶▶ Vitamin C prevents the secretion of histamine by white blood cells.

▶▶ Vitamin C (1,000 mg per day) detoxifies excess histamine (by converting histamine to hydantoin-5-acetic acid, which then decomposes into metabolic by-products for excretion).

▶▶ Vitamin C facilitates the urinary excretion of excessive uric acid from the body.

▶▶ Vitamin C counteracts the lung damage caused by exposure to nitrogen oxides (especially from exposure to nitrogen dioxide, a component of air pollution).

▶▶ Vitamin C lowers elevated fibrinogen levels, and elevated fibrinogen levels can occur as a result of vitamin C deficiency. (Elevated fibrinogen is implicated in abnormal blood clotting.)

▶▶ Vitamin C (especially when combined with cysteine and vitamin B1) reduces the toxicity of alcohol.

▶▶ Vitamin C accelerates the clearance of alcohol from the blood plasma.

Vitamin C (if consumed at the same time as consuming alcoholic beverages) helps to prevent hangovers.

▶▶ Alcoholics are generally found to be deficient in vitamin C and vitamin C accelerates the clearance of alcohol from the blood plasma.

▶▶ Vitamin C reduces the withdrawal symptoms associated with drug dependence caused by heroin.

▶▶ Vitamin C counteracts some of the toxic effects associated with tobacco smoking and reduces the toxic effects of nicotine.

▶▶ Vitamin C improves the function of the endothelium in tobacco smokers (and thereby helps to prevent atherosclerosis in tobacco smokers).

Selenium

Selenium is a trace mineral that is essential to good health in small amounts. Selenium is incorporated into proteins to make selenoproteins, which are important antioxidant enzymes. The antioxidant properties of selenoproteins help prevent cellular damage from free radicals. Free radicals are natural by-products of oxygen metabolism that may contribute to the development of chronic diseases such as cancer and heart disease. Other selenoproteins help regulate thyroid function and play a role in the immune system.

- Selenium enhances the function of cysteine.
- Selenium is an essential element of the glutathione synthase enzyme.
- Selenium is a cofactor for the production of superoxide dismutase (SOD).
- Selenium mimics the actions of insulin.
- Low testosterone levels (in males) can occur as a result of selenium deficiency.
- Selenium alleviates the chest pain associated with angina, and angina can occur as a result of selenium deficiency.
- Selenium helps to prevent atherosclerosis.
- Crohn's disease patients commonly exhibit abnormally low selenium levels.
- Selenium is required for the proper function of the pancreas.
- Chronic pancreatitis patients have low blood selenium levels (indicating that supplemental selenium may prevent or alleviate pancreatitis).
- Selenium alleviates euthyroid sick syndrome due to its role as cofactor for 5'-deiodinase (type 1), which catalyzes the conversion of thyroxine to triiodothyronine in peripheral tissues.

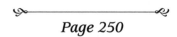

- Selenium is useful for the treatment of hypothyroidism (due to its role in the conversion of thyroxine (T4) to triiodothyronine (T3).
- Selenium helps to lower elevated blood sugar levels in diabetes mellitus patients.
- Selenium maintains and improves the function of the liver.
- Alzheimer's disease patients are generally found to be deficient in selenium.
- Selenium deficiency can cause anxiety in patients.
- Multiple sclerosis (MS) patients generally have low selenium levels (indicating that supplemental selenium may be beneficial for MS patients).
- Selenium may be useful for the treatment of asthma.

L-carnosine

L-carnosine is a dipeptide composed of the amino acids beta-alanine and L-histidine. L-carnosine is a naturally occurring amino acid found in high concentrations in muscle, heart, and brain tissues. L-carnosine — not to be confused with the popular supplement, L-carnitine — is a highly effective anti-aging nutrient that possesses powerful antioxidant, free radical scavenging, and neurotransmitter properties. Carnosine inhibits the formation of carbonyl groups, thereby reducing the formation of abnormal proteins. L-carnosine extends maximum cell division capacity, protects against DNA oxidation, blocks glycosylation, and reduces advanced glycation end products (AGEs), as well as acting as a cell membrane stabilizer and an intracellular buffer.

L-carnosine is already a well-established anti-aging nutrient that is used to treat liver disease, cataracts, Alzheimer's disease, and cancer. L-carnosine has recently been shown to possess a tremendous potential for improving language and behavior in children diagnosed with autistic spectrum disorders (ASD).

Health benefits of carnosine

Carnosine retards some aspects of the aging process. (Specifically, it maintains the defense mechanisms of fibroblasts, inhibits cross-linking, and improves the efficiency of the synthesis of endogenous proteins.) The body's levels of carnosine decline by up to 63% in tandem with the progression of the aging process.

▸▸ Carnosine helps to prevent (chemical-induced) hemolytic anemia (by stabilizing the cell membranes of red blood cells).

▸▸ Carnosine helps to prevent abnormal blood clotting (by reducing platelet aggregation).

▸▸ Carnosine functions as an antioxidant in cell membranes and prevents lipid peroxidation within cell membranes.

▸▸ Carnosine helps to prevent gastric ulcers and accelerates the healing of gastric ulcers.

▸▸ Carnosine helps to prevent cancer and may facilitate the regression of some types of cancer. (It inhibits the process of glycolysis in cancer cells — cancer cells are highly dependent upon glycolysis to meet their requirement for the energy that helps them to grow and replicate.)

▸▸ Carnosine stimulates the immune system by activating B-lymphocytes and T-lymphocytes, increases the production of interleukin 1 by neutrophils, and enhances the function of neutrophils.

▸▸ Carnosine reduces inflammation.

▸▸ Carnosine quenches hydroxyl, peroxyl, singlet oxygen, and superoxide free radicals.

▸▸ Carnosine prevents the cross-linking of endogenous proteins and blocks the production of advanced glycosylation end-products (AGEs) and carbonylated proteins that are formed as a result of cross-linking. Also, carnosine interacts with and deactivates various aldehydes and ketones that initiate the process of cross-linking and which initiate the formation of advanced glycosylation end-products (AGEs).

▸▸ Carnosine enhances the ability of macrophages to recognize and eliminate advanced glycosylation end-products (AGEs).

▸▸ Carnosine protects the brain against the toxic effects of ischemia.

▸▸ Carnosine enhances the performance of people who undertake isotonic exercise (i.e. weight lifting).

▸▸ Carnosine helps to protect the liver from the effects of various toxins (including carbon tetrachloride).

▸▸ Carnosine helps to rejuvenate connective tissue cells.

▸▸ Carnosine concentrates in skeletal muscle.

▸▸ Carnosine blocks and inactivates amyloid-beta protein and prevents the cell damage caused by amyloid-beta protein. Carnosine also inhibits the cross-linking of amyloid-beta protein that leads to the formation of the senile plaques in the brains of Alzheimer's disease patients.

▸▸ Carnosine concentrates in the brain (where it helps to counteract excitotoxicity and the toxic effects of copper and zinc in the brain). It also helps to protect the brain against the toxic effects of ischemia.

▸▸ Carnosine maintains the defense mechanisms of fibroblasts and inhibits oxidative damage to fibroblasts.

My personal Detox formula

This formula contains all necessary amino acids and nutrients for detoxification.

▸▸ Promotes healthy liver function and promotes healthy GI function.

▸▸ Provides adjunctive support for weight loss by supporting healthy insulin function and inhibition of carbohydrate and fat calorie absorption, and support for stage 1 P450 and stage 2 of detoxification of liver.

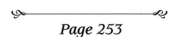

➤ Enhances kidney function by stimulating the regeneration of the kidneys and protects the kidneys from the toxic effects of many toxins.

➤ Lowers cholesterol and LDL, and increases HDL.

➤ Supports immune functions.

➤ Supports lung functions by preventing damage to the lungs from free radicals and environmental ozone.

➤ Reverses abnormal blood clotting.

➤ Dosage: Two capsules three times/day with meals

Qurceplex: quercetin and bromelain

Quercetin is the most abundant of the flavonoids. Quercetin is also a building block for other flavonoids. Quercetin is found in many common foods including apple, tea, onion, nuts, berries, cauliflower, and cabbage.

Action of quercetin: includes improvement of cardiovascular health and reducing risk for cancer. Quercetin has anti-inflammatory and anti-allergic effects. The anti-inflammatory action of quercetin is caused by the inhibition of enzymes, such as lipoxygenase, and the inhibition of inflammatory mediators.

Quercetin also inhibits the release of histamine, which causes congestion, by basophiles and mast cells and prevents the depletion of glutathione from the cells of the intestinal tract.

Quercetin increases mucus secretion from gastric cells. The mucus polysaccharide provides a protective buffer for the gastric cells from the low pH of the stomach contents. The reduced contact provides protection from gastric lesions.

Activated quercetin with bromelain is a unique bioflavonoid which makes more potent antioxidants, and bromelain increases the absorption of quercetin. Bromelain is a proteolytic enzyme from the pineapple plant. It is functional throughout a wide pH range and does not lose its activity as it goes through the acidic environment of the stomach.

Dosage: Two capsules two times/day with meals

L-phenylalanine

L-phenylalanine is a protein amino acid. It is classified as an essential amino acid because the body requires a dietary source of the amino acid to meet its physiological demands. L-phenylalanine is found in proteins of all life forms. Dietary sources of the amino acid are principally derived from animal and vegetable proteins. Vegetables and juices contain small amounts of the free amino acid. Phenylalanine suppresses appetite (by stimulating the production of cholecystokinin hormone). Phenylalanine is involved in the production of collagen. L-phenylalanine can be converted to L-tyrosine, which takes place in the liver. L-tyrosine can be converted by neurons in the brain to dopamine and norepinephrine (noradrenaline), which is mental energy. Those hormones get depleted by stress, use of certain drugs, and lack of nutrients. Cells in the adrenal medulla synthesize and secrete norepinephrine and epinephrine from L-tyrosine with cofactors (vitamins B6 and C). Norepinephrine and epinephrine can cause smooth muscle (arterial) contraction. People with blood pressure should be careful when they take L-phenylalanine or L-tyrosine.

Caffeine lowers plasma phenylalanine levels.

Dosage: One capsule one time/day before breakfast

Multi-probiotic

Probiotic is one of the factors for our health. Various species of beneficial bacteria (as well as various species of potentially detrimental bacteria) populate the colon. Beneficial bacteria in the colon convert cholesterol to coprostanol for excretion, thereby lowering total serum cholesterol levels. Beneficial bacteria strengthen the immune system functions of the intestines.

Beneficial bacteria alleviate some of the symptoms of irritable bowel syndrome (especially intestinal cramps [abdominal pain] and flatulence).

Beneficial bacteria enhance the function of the immune system.

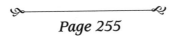

(By producing substances such as acetic acid, bacteriocins, lactic acid, and hydrogen peroxide, beneficial bacteria help to counteract antigens such as detrimental bacteria and viruses.)

Dosage: Two capsules with dinner

EDTA (ethylenediamine tetra-acetic acid)

EDTA was proposed in the late 1950's for removal of calcium from atherosclerotic plaques. EDTA is a man-made amino acid primarily used as a chelating agent in chelation therapy. EDTA removes toxic metals from the blood. Studies have shown that as people age, they continuously accumulate toxic metals: lead, mercury, aluminum, iron, cadmium, and arsenic, among others. The accrual of these toxins invites an increased risk for various diseases, especially heart disease. The less of these metals we have in our bodies, the more likely we are to be physiologically healthy or simply feel good, and the lower our risk for heart disease.

Dosage: Two capsules three times/day with meals

Cholesterol formula

This formula promotes healthy liver function, maintains optimal healthy cholesterol, and supports and maintains ideal HDL/LDL ratios, all of which aid in normalizing elevated lipids and help to decrease triglyceride. The cholesterol formula promotes healthy cholesterol levels — whether you've already been diagnosed with high cholesterol or just want to prevent future problems. Diet and exercise are one part of the solution. Your age, stress, poor eating habits, and genetics are all factors that over time cause the cholesterol and fats in your bloodstream (triglycerides) to continue to accumulate. The cholesterol formula provides a powerful combination of ingredients to help decrease your high cholesterol. The cholesterol formula, an all-natural formula, decreases

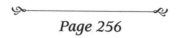

cholesterol and LDL (low density lipoprotein) and increases HDL (high density lipoprotein).

Dosage: Two capsules three times/day with meals

Multi-vitamin (men and women)

Do we need multi-vitamins?

This is the question everybody asks, and my response is, "Are you healthy, and do you eat healthy?" Healthy eating includes consuming fresh vegetables, complex carbohydrates, wild fish, and fruits. If you do, then you might think you don't need to take vitamins. Even if you eat well, the food doesn't have enough of the nutrients that your body needs. You can be vitamin D deficient if you suffer from lactose intolerance — the physical symptoms of intestinal gas, cramps, diarrhea, and bloating when you consume milk or other dairy products. People over age 50 can become B12 deficient due to hypochlorhydria (low acid in stomach) and cannot digest their food. Now you make the choice to take a multi-vitamin or not.

I created a multi-vitamin for myself and my family, since I could not find a good quality multi-vitamin in the market. Most once-a-day multi-vitamins contain dosages at the Recommended Daily Allowance (RDA) levels designed to merely prevent deficiencies of vitamins and minerals. The usual multi-vitamins at RDA levels are believed to have little or no effect on health or on our longevity, and RDA levels were never designed for optimal health maintenance. I do know from my own clinical experience that taking a high-quality multi-vitamin with moderately high dosages of nutrients is necessary for your health. In addition, nutritional supplements from capsules are better absorbed by the body. Take the supplements to prevent diseases. In the society we live in, almost everyone has a family history that includes a chronic illness such as heart disease, high cholesterol, diabetes, or cancer. You may be concerned that you carry a genetic predisposition to one or more of these diseases; we can help prevent them, and recent science has shown there's much we can do, starting with nutrition.

Multi-vitamins help all our organs function better. This multi-vitamin supplies the whole list of essential vitamins including A, B complex, C, D, and E in a natural form and supplies the important minerals including calcium, magnesium, chromium, potassium, selenium, zinc, manganese, and amino acid. They support physical and mental energy that helps keep you mentally alert and focused, with a better mood and more energized and motivated, and perhaps you even get more work done during the day.

Dosage: You can take up to nine capsules/day with meals, depending on your daily work load.

Glucoton

Glucoton helps maintain optimal blood sugar, supports and maintains energy, aids in normalizing elevated sugar, and helps balance the energy of cells. It also maintains a healthy liver to reduce fat production and maintains and supports a healthy pancreas and maximized insulin usage.

Dosage: Two capsules three times/day with meals

Ginkgo biloba

Ginkgo biloba is one of the most effective known substances for enhancing blood circulation to the capillaries, and ginkgo biloba alleviates cerebral insufficiency, which helps with memory. Ginkgo biloba may counteract the aging process.

Dosage: Two capsules between meals

L-tyrosine

L-tyrosine is a non-essential amino acid that the body synthesizes

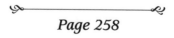

from phenylalanine and another amino acid. Tyrosine is important to the structure of almost all proteins in the body. It is also the precursor of several neurotransmitters, including L-dopa, dopamine, norepinephrine, and epinephrine. L-tyrosine may affect several health conditions, including depression, Parkinson's disease, and other mood disorders.

▶ L-tyrosine normalizes blood pressure in some hypotension patients.

▶ Tyrosine inhibits further hair loss (but only when hair loss is caused by hypothyroidism).

▶ Tyrosine increases the body's production of energy (by stimulating the thyroid gland and by facilitating the production of norepinephrine).

▶ Tyrosine indirectly increases energy levels in some chronic fatigue syndrome patients (by increasing the brain's production of norepinephrine).

▶ Tyrosine stimulates weight loss in persons who are afflicted with obesity (but only when obesity is due to hypothyroidism). The underlying mechanism for this effect is tyrosine's role in the production of thyroid hormones.

▶ Tyrosine alleviates excessive stress on the adrenal glands (due to its function as a precursor for the endogenous production of adrenaline).

Caution: Tyrosine should not be used by patients with hyperthyroidism. Persons with blood pressure should be careful when they take L-phenylalanine or L-tyrosine.

Dosage: One capsule before breakfast on an empty stomach

Osteo-support

It is estimated that over 25 million adults in the United States have, or are at risk of developing, osteoporosis, which results in 1.5 million fractures each year, mostly in the spine, hip, or wrist. To support healthy bones and bone loss, this formula prevents osteoporosis by activating calcitonin and by inhibiting osteoclasts and enabling calcitonin to transfer calcium into the bones. This formula is designed to help prevent tooth decay and osteoporosis by protecting your bones against brittleness and deterioration. It contains calcium and is fortified with vitamin D3, vitamin K1, magnesium, and other bone-strengthening minerals that are difficult to obtain in a regular diet. Osteoporosis is a disease that attacks and weakens bones, and half the women alive today are at increased risk of developing osteoporosis by the age 50.

Dosage: Two capsules two times/day with meals

Betaine plus

Betaine hydrochloride is recommended for people who have a deficiency of stomach acid production (hypochlorhydria). A deficiency of gastric acid secretion increases the likelihood and severity of certain bacterial and parasitic intestinal infections. A normal stomach's level of gastric acid is sufficient to destroy bacteria. Betaine hydrochloride alleviates many cases of heartburn (by increasing the level of hydrochloric acid in the stomach). Betaine increases the liver's efficiency in metabolizing fatty acids. Betaine reduces homocysteine levels. During its metabolism within the body, betaine transfers one of its methyl groups to homocysteine, causing homocysteine to be converted to methionine. Betaine helps to prevent cirrhosis and also helps to prevent and reverse fatty liver. Children, women who are pregnant, and nursing mothers should not take betaine HCL because it is not really known if it is safe for them.

Dosage: One capsule with non-meats, two capsules with white meat, and three capsules with red meat

7-keto (DHEA)

7-keto (3-acetyl 7-oxo-dehydroepiandrosterone) is a naturally

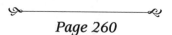

occurring metabolite (breakdown product) of the hormone dehydroepiandrosterone (DHEA), and DHEA is synthesized primarily in the adrenal glands from the steroid precursor pregnenolone, which is synthesized from cholesterol. DHEA is the main precursor for estradiol and testosterone. In the blood, most DHEA is sulfated (DHEA-S04), providing a storage depot for DHEA, thereby prolonging its half life and providing a steady state source of DHEA for conversion to estrogens and androgens in the adrenal glands, ovaries, and testes.

7-keto DHEA is very similar to DHEA. The primary difference between 7-keto DHEA and regular DHEA is that the anabolic properties of DHEA are maximized while the androgenic effects (which are problematic) are minimized with 7-keto DHEA. There are also claims that 7-keto DHEA is more potent in terms of therapeutic effects compared to regular DHEA. Unlike regular DHEA, 7-keto DHEA is NOT transformed into testosterone or estrogens.

Weight gain is a common sign of decreased DHEA and its metabolites, and its levels decrease with age. 7-keto accelerates the loss of body fat while maintaining muscle tissue integrity to help maintain healthy body weight (by facilitating thermogenesis).

7-keto supports proper immune, response, mental well-being, thyroid functions, and vascular health.

Dosage: One capsules one time/day at 10 am

L-lysine

Lysine is one of nine essential amino acids that the body needs for growth and tissue repair.

Lack of lysine in the diet, kidney stones, and other health related problems may develop including fatigue, nausea, dizziness, loss of appetite, agitation, bloodshot eyes, slow growth, anemia, and reproductive disorders.

▸▸ Lysine helps to prevent kidney stones (by preventing the

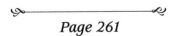

excretion of calcium — a component of calcium oxalate kidney stones — in the urine).

▸▸ Lysine stimulates the production of antibodies and accelerates the healing of the lesions associated with herpes simplex viruses.

▸▸ Hair loss can occur as a result of lysine deficiency.

▸▸ Lysine helps to prevent osteoporosis by enhancing the absorption and utilization of calcium.

Dosage: One capsule two times/day between meals

Sleep formula

This formula helps to maintain optimal sleep by increasing melatonin and aids in normalizing elevated serotonin, which also helps with mood swings. It also supports and maintains energy, maintains younger looking skin with a good night's sleep, and also supports the immune system.

Dosage: Two capsules ½ hour before bed

Phyto cleanse

This is used to alleviate constipation and regulate bowel movements, normalization, gastrointestinal motility, vitality, and also supports the immune system.

Dosage: One to two capsules with dinner

EPA/DHA (fish oil) PCB/heavy metal free

Most of the health benefits associated with fish oils are attributable to both docosahexaenoic acid (DHA) and eicosapentaenoic acid (EPA); most nut oils and vegetable oils contain alpha-linolenic acid (ALA). Fish oil is necessary for the production of anti-inflammatory prostaglandins (E1 and E3) and helps lower the body's production of prostaglandin E2.

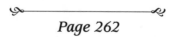

Regular consumption of fish oils helps to prevent autoimmune diseases, breast cancer, colon cancer, lung cancer, pancreatic cancer, and prostate cancer.

- ▸▸ Fish oils help to suppress inflammation (due to the DHA and EPA content of fish oils).
- ▸▸ Fish oils reduce the absorption of dietary cholesterol and reduce the synthesis of cholesterol within the liver.
- ▸▸ Fish oils increase insulin sensitivity in insulin-resistant patients and help to prevent insulin resistance.

Dosage: Two capsules two times/day with meals

Vitamin D3

The major biologic function of vitamin D3 is to maintain normal blood levels of calcium and phosphorus. Vitamin D3 aids in the absorption of calcium, helping to form and maintain strong bones. Recently, research also suggests vitamin D3 may provide protection from osteoporosis, hypertension, breast cancer, prostate cancer, depression, and several autoimmune diseases. Vitamin D3 is perhaps the single most under-rated nutrient in the world of nutrition. Vitamin D3 deficiency can also result in tooth decay, weak muscles, pain in the bones, and muscle spasms.

Vitamin D3 is a steroid hormone precursor that plays a role in a wide variety of diseases.

Vitamin D3 is one of the several forms of vitamin D — functionally, vitamin D3 (cholecalciferol) is a pre-hormone that has long been known for its important role in regulating body levels of calcium and phosphorus, and in mineralization of bone. Vitamin D3 activates osteoblasts, which prevent osteoporosis.

Dosage: One tablet two times/day with meals

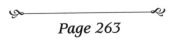

Digestive Enzyme

Digestive enzymes alleviate heartburn and indigestion by facilitating the digestion of undigested food in the stomach that may be causing heartburn and indigestion. The principal digestive enzymes used to treat heartburn include:
- Amylase (which digests polysaccharides)
- Cellulose (which digests cellulose)
- Lipases (which digest dietary fats)
- Proteolytic enzymes (which digest dietary proteins)

Supplemental digestive enzymes alleviate indigestion (by facilitating the digestion of undigested food in the stomach that may be causing indigestion).
Dosage: Two capsules two times/day with meals

Black cohosh

(Botanical name has recently been renamed from cimicifuge racemosa.)

Black cohosh is popular as an alternative to hormonal therapy in the treatment of menopausal (climacteric) symptoms such as hot flashes, mood disturbances, diaphoresis, palpitations, depression, vaginal dryness, and vaginal atrophy commonly experienced by menopausal women.

Black cohosh alleviates many of the symptoms of female menopause (due to the 27-deoxyacteine content of black cohosh).
Dosage: Two capsules one time/day with breakfast

Indinol (Indole-3-carbinol)

Indinol is primarily found in cruciferous vegetables (cabbage, broccoli sprouts, Brussels sprouts, cauliflower, bok choy, and kale). Indole-3-carbinol may modulate estrogen metabolism. It may also have anticarcinogenic, antioxidant, and anti-atherogenic activities.

Indole-3-carbinol inhibits the conversion of estrone to 16-hydroxyestrone (a carcinogenic metabolite of estrone) and redirects estrone to be converted to 2-hydroxyestrone (a safe metabolite of estrone), keeping balanced estrogen.

Indole-3-carbinol is a strong antioxidant and stimulator of detoxifying enzymes. Indole-3-carbinol seems to protect the structure of DNA. Indole-3-carbinol blocks estrogen receptor sites on the membranes of breast and other cells, thereby reducing the risk of breast and cervical cancer.

Indole-3-carbinol stimulates the conversion of estrone to its inactive (safe) metabolite, 2-hydroxyestrone, and inhibits the conversion of estrone to its carcinogenic metabolite, 16-hydroxyestrone. The estrogen metabolite 2-hydroxyestrone has been protective against several types of cancer and dioxin. It may alleviate some of the symptoms of chronic fatigue syndrome (CFS) and fibromyalgia.

Indole-3-carbinol should not be used by women during pregnancy (due to its effects on estrogen).

Dosage: One capsule one time/day without meal

Hair, skin, and nails

This formula is designed to provide optimal support for healthier hair, skin and nails. It has the beneficial vitamins of A and C, which have powerful antioxidant properties that protect the cells from daily environmental damage. Other ingredients , such as horsetail grass, help to repair and maintain delicate connective tissue.

Dosage: Two capsules two times/day with meals

L-glutamine

L-glutamine is the most abundant amino acid in the body muscle cells, and plasma glutamine levels are the highest of any

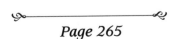

amino acid. L-glutamine is predominantly synthesized and stored in skeletal muscle. The amino acid L-glutamate is metabolized to L-glutamine in a reaction catalyzed by the enzyme glutamine synthase, a reaction which, in addition to L-glutamate, requires ammonia, ATP, and magnesium. L-glutamine is lost from muscle during times of stress, heavy weight training, workouts, and dieting. This amino acid not only has been shown to be a great anti-catabolic agent (protects the muscle from the catabolic activities of the hormone cortisol), to be a contributor to muscle cell volume, and to have immune system enhancing properties, but it also helps in the regulation of protein synthesis, which is used in muscle building .

Glutamine is in high demand throughout the body. It is used in the gut and immune system extensively to maintain optimal performance.

L-glutamine helps control the negative biochemical effects resulting from the build-up of the waste by-products resulting from hard exercise. Glutamine functions as a nitrogen shuttle — it "picks up and drops off" nitrogen around the body. Glutamine facilitates the elimination of ammonia from the body. Stress causes severe depletion of glutamine.

L-glutamine reduces body weight in persons afflicted with obesity (by approximately 10%). L-glutamine reduces cravings for simple sugars. L-glutamine supplementation increases the production of arginine (in the kidneys).

Dosage: Two capsules two times/day with meals

Prostrate Health

The active ingredients of Prostrate Health have been shown to positively affect the structure and function of the prostate gland during the normal aging of men. Saw Palmetto (Serenoa repens), aided by pygeum (Pygeum africanum), inhibits the conversion of testosterone to its more active, and potentially deleterious form, dihydrotestosterone (DHT), via inhibition of alpha-5- reductase. Saw palmetto not only inhibits the binding of DHT to cellular receptors, but also has alpha1-adrenoceptor-inhibitory properties. Alpha1- adrenoceptor antagonism may be responsible for saw palmetto's therapeutic effect in supporting the urinary tract during the normal aging of men. Saw palmetto extracts have also been found to inhibit the biosynthesis of proinflammatory prostaglandins and leukotrienes which may exacerbate those symptoms. Supplementation with Pygeum africanum extract, in men 50 to 75 years, significantly improved several aspects of prostate function, including nocturnal frequency, maximum flow and volume. Pygeum extract decreases prolactin and cholesterol levels in the prostate, which in turn decreases uptake and reduces the number of binding sites for testosterone in the prostate. In addition, pygeum extract, like saw palmetto, interferes with the synthesis of proinflammatory prostaglandins. Pumpkin seed is thought to have similar pharmacotherapeutic properties. Vitamin E, zinc, and proanthocyanidins provide potent antioxidant protection against oxidative damage to the prostate. The amino acids glycine, alanine, and glutamic acid, as well as vitamin B-6 and vitamin A, have been suggested to reduce proliferation of prostate tissue cells.

Dosage: One capsule two times/day without meals

Methylcobalamin drops, vitamin B12 liquid drops

Vitamin B12 is a member of the vitamin B complex. It contains cobalt, and so is also known as cobalamin. It is exclusively synthesized by bacteria and is found primarily in meat, eggs, and dairy products.

Vitamin B12 is an essential water-soluble vitamin that is commonly found in a variety of foods such as fish, shellfish, meats, and dairy products. Vitamin B12 is frequently used in combination

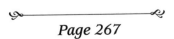

with other B vitamins in a vitamin B complex formulation. It helps maintain healthy nerve cells and red blood cells and is also needed to make DNA, the genetic material in all cells. Vitamin B12 is bound to the protein in food. Hydrochloric acid in the stomach releases B12 from protein during digestion. Once released, B12 combines with a substance called intrinsic factor (IF) before it is absorbed into the bloodstream. Vitamin B12 is essential for the formation of red blood cells. Vitamin B12 deficiency contributes to hypochlorhydria (low acidity of the stomach). Vitamin B12 is important for the normal functioning of the brain and nervous system. The methylcobalamin form of vitamin B12 helps to prevent the damage to neurons caused by exposure to excessive levels of glutamic acid.

Vitamin B12 is responsible for red blood cell formation. Vitamin B12 lowers elevated homocysteine levels by functioning as a cofactor for the methionine synthase enzyme that catalyzes the conversion (remethylation) of homocysteine to form methionine. (Excessive homocysteine is a risk factor for many cardiovascular diseases.)

Dosage: 10 drops under tongue daily

Vital kids immune support

The immune system is the body's defense against infectious organisms and other invaders. Children are prone to infectious diseases when the immune system isn't functioning properly. The key to a healthy child is a strong immune system. When the immune system is strong, it will fight disease-producing organisms such as bacteria, viruses, fungi, and parasites. All children are continuously exposed to these pathogens, but exposure does not mean a child will get sick. A strong immune system provides a child with powerful natural defenses against disease. Vital kids immune support helps the immune system to support their bodies against those infectious diseases.

Dosage: As directed

Glucosamine + MSM formula

Glucosamine is a small molecule; it is easily absorbed and very permeable to cell linings. Glucosamine with MSM causes healthier joints and pain relief due to the MSM, which enhances the health of the body's cartilage and also the formation of cartilage (by contributing its sulfur content to cartilage), without the side effects.

MSM is a naturally occurring sulfur compound found in the tissues and fluids of all living organisms. It is naturally found in raw unprocessed milk, meat, fish, fruits, and vegetables. Most of the usable MSM is lost during washing and cooking. Also, food processing companies deplete the food from sulfur, which we need, during packaging and preparation.

Dosage: Two capsules two times/day with meals

Children's (multi-vitamin)

Children who are picky eaters and enjoy too much junk food, including school lunches, or live in households where their meals are convenience-type meals (from frozen food or microwave food), do not get enough vitamins and minerals. These children should be taking vitamin supplements. Children also need some extra daily vitamin C to support their immune systems.

Dosage: Two capsules two times/day with meals

Flaxseed oil

Flaxseed oil and flaxseed contain substances that promote good health. Flaxseed is one-third oil and the rest is made up of fiber. Flaxseed oil is rich in alpha-linolenic acid (ALA), an essential fatty acid, protein, and mucilage, and also a great source of a group of chemicals called lignans that appear to be beneficial for heart disease, inflammatory bowel disease, arthritis, and a variety of other health conditions. Lignans may also play a role in the prevention of cancer.

Dosage: Two capsules two times/day with meals

Brain support

Phosphatidylserine (PS) is a phosphoglyceride phospholipid that occurs naturally in the brain, and PS deficiency is common with age. PS restocks brain cell membranes, boosting nerve chemical activity such as dopamine and serotonin, stimulating nerve cell growth, lowering levels of the stress hormones, possibly generating new connections between cells, and stirring activity in all brain centers, especially higher brain centers such as the cortex, hypothalamus, and pituitary gland. Phosphatidylserine facilitates the production and release of acetylcholine within the cerebral cortex and reverses the decline in acetylcholine release that occurs in tandem with the progression of the aging process. Phosphatidylserine enhances the efficiency of glucose metabolism within the brain.

Dosage: One capsule two times/day without meals

Co Qenzyme10 (ubiquinol)

Coenzyme Q10 exists in both ubiquinol and ubiquinone forms, but they have very different roles to play in the body. When it comes to choosing a CoQ10 supplement, the best form is ubiquinol, the reduced (active) form of CoQ10, the form which is directly used in human metabolism as a lipid-soluble antioxidant. Scientific studies show that ubiquinol absorbs up to eight times greater than ubiquinone and that higher levels of ubiquinol remain in the blood far longer than ubiquinone. In recent studies measuring exercise-induced fatigue, ubiquinol was 90% more effective than ubiquinone. In middle-aged mice, ubiquinol was shown to be 40% more effective in slowing measurements of aging compared to ubiquinone. Coenzyme Q10 is a component of almost every cell of the body. Coenzyme Q10 has been found to reverse accelerated abnormal apoptosis of cells involved in the aging process. Coenzyme Q10 increases the production of energy within the mitochondria of cells and increases oxygen supplies to the mitochondria — the mitochondrion contains approximately 50% of the body's total coenzyme Q10 content. Coenzyme Q10 also functions as an antioxidant. People with statin drug (cholesterol drug) lose 30 to 40% of their coenzyme Q10 from their body, therefore supplementation of coenzyme Q10 is necessary for those patients.

Dosage: Two capsules one time/day with meal

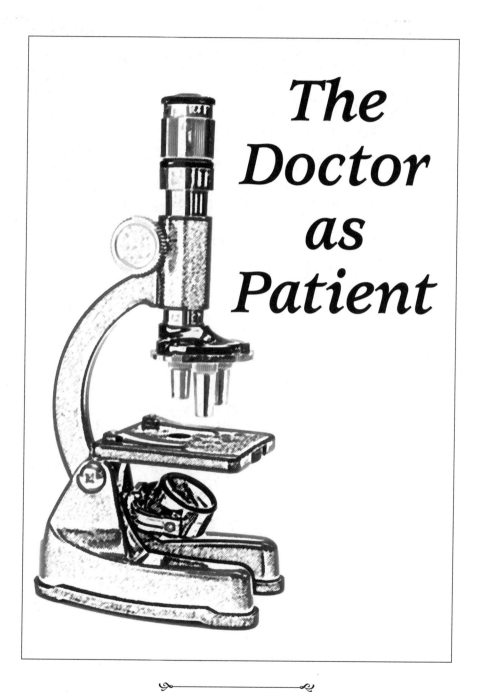

The Doctor as Patient

The Doctor as Patient

To prove to my patients, and to you the reader, I spent several weeks eating all the things that I normally say "no" to. You can refer back to page 187 to read what I did. Below is my before and after blood work. It did not take long for my body chemistry to go haywire as indicated in the values of my glucose and cholesterol. However it was all fixable, once I went through detox and went back to living the life style I am suggesting in these pages.

Lab results for Dr. Sokhandan from PACLAB in Everett, Washington before going on detox:

	Value	Reference Range
Glucose	89	65-114 mg/dL
CRP Non-Cardiac	1.0	0.0-7.9 mg/dL
Cholesterol	214	0-199 mg/dL
HDL	39	40-59 mg/dL
LDL Direct	151	< =99 mg/dL
A1C	6.1	4.0-6.0 %
TSH	1.56	0.4-5 uIU/mL
Estradiol II	38	8-43 pg/mL
DHEA-SO4	370	58-257 ug/dL
Vitamin D 25 Hydroxy	27	30-150 ng/mL

Lab results for Dr. Sokhandan from PACLAB in Everett, Washington after four weeks on detox:

	Value	Reference Range
Glucose	69	65-114 mg/dL
CRP Non-Cardiac	0.4	0.0-7.9 mg/dL
Cholesterol	160	0-199 mg/dL
HDL	38	40-59 mg/dL
LDL Direct	105	< =99 mg/dL

A1C...5.5.................................4.0-6.0 %
TSH...................................... 1.56...................... 0.4-5 uIU/mL
Estradiol II ....38 .... 8-43 pg/mL
DHEA-SO4.............................value 307 reference range 58-257 ug/dL
Vitamin D 25 Hydroxy............value 54reference range 30-150 ng/mL

For people without diabetes blood sugar levels should be between 70 and 120 mg/ dL. Although I was not in danger of becoming a diabetic during my experiment, my glucose did change by 20 points. However had I stayed on my course of bad eating habits I have no doubt I would have become diabetic over time.

The Cardio CRP® blood test included in this report is a measure of vascular inflammation, which can be a strong indicator of future cardiovascular disease. Once again you can see that the detox lowered this value to a extremely safe range.

Cholesterol, which is found in foods high in saturated fat, is necessary for the structure and functioning of our cells. However, to much cholesterol in your blood will lead to a buildup of plaque in the arteries. LDL is the, so called, bad cholesterol and HDL is the good cholesterol because it assists in returning cholesterol back to the liver where it can be dumped by the body.

The A1C test (also known as HbA1C test or glycated hemoglobin test) provides a long-term look at blood sugar control. It is a sample of hemoglobin A1C cells—a specific component of your red blood cells.

The TSH test is often the test of choice for evaluating thyroid function and/or symptoms of hyper- or hypothyroidism. It is frequently ordered along with or preceding a T4 test. Other thyroid tests that may be ordered include a T3 test and thyroid antibodies (if autoimmune-related thyroid disease is suspected).

The TSH can let a person know how well their thyroid is functioning and the Estradiol II is a hormone that plays a key role in your mood. The function of your adrenal gland is determined with the DHEAS-S04 levels.

Finally Vitamin D is important as it is a key element in determining the strength of your immune system.

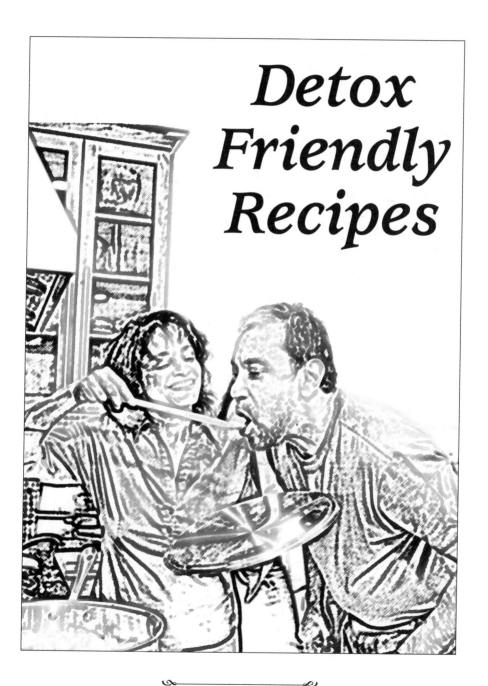

Detox Friendly Recipes

Detox friendly recipes

DAY 1
Breakfast: Organic steel-cut oats with a dash of soy milk and a sprinkle of cinnamon. Add fresh fruit if you like or add fruit-juice-sweetened jam to the oatmeal to make it sweet.

Lunch: Spicy chicken chili with salad *(see recipe)*.

Snacks: Carrot sticks, rye crisps, brown rice cakes with almond butter and fruit-juice-sweetened jam, organic almonds, apple slices, or other fruits as permitted.

Dinner: Grilled chicken with grilled potatoes — use your choice of spices and herbs like dill and garlic, with sea salt and/or pepper.
Serve with sliced tomatoes with a light sprinkle of sea salt.

DAY 2
Breakfast: Spelt or rye bread with almond butter and fruit-juice-sweetened jam.

Lunch: Chicken fajita salad (see recipe) with a little green chili sauce *(see recipe)*.

Snacks: Carrot sticks, rye crisps, brown rice cakes with almond butter and fruit-juice-sweetened jam, organic almonds, apple slices.

Dinner: Spaghetti with organic brown rice noodles *(see spaghetti sauce recipe)* and salad.

DAY 3
Breakfast: Fruit smoothie *(see recipe)*.

Lunch: Chicken wild rice soup *(see recipe)*.

Snacks: Carrot sticks, rye crisps, brown rice cakes with almond butter and fruit-juice-sweetened jam, organic almonds, apple slices.

Dinner: Grill up your favorite fresh fish (salmon) with grilled asparagus or steamed carrots.

RECIPES

When cooking recipes, try to cook with all organic ingredients.

Fruit Smoothie

RECIPE INGREDIENTS
- 1 cup organic unsweetened soy milk
- 1 medium organic apple, cut into chunks and frozen
- 1/2 cup of your favorite fruit, frozen (peaches, pitted cherries, blueberries, blackberries, mango, etc.)
- 2 tablespoons organic almond butter (if desired for protein)

DIRECTIONS
Place all ingredients in a blender and purée until smooth.

Spelt Pancakes

Whole grain pancakes are a great way to start your morning! This recipe can be easily doubled.

Spelt is an ancient form of wheat. It contains more protein, fiber, and vitamins than wheat. It has a nutty flavor and is slightly heavier than whole wheat.

Preparation time: 5 minutes
Cooking time: 10-12 minutes
Makes: 4 pancakes
Preheat pancake griddle.

RECIPE INGREDIENTS
- 1 cup spelt flour
- 1 ¼ cup unsweetened organic soy milk
- 2 egg whites, beaten
- 2 tablespoons grape seed oil (to grease pancake griddle)
- 1 tablespoon grape seed (for pancake batter)

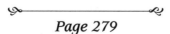

◀ 1 teaspoon baking powder (aluminum free)

Serve with a fresh strawberry puree or fruit-juice-sweetened jam with almond butter.

Breakfast Wrap

This hearty breakfast wrap is full of protein to give you balanced energy. You can also use spelt or brown rice tortillas. Use organic ingredients wherever possible.

Preparation time: 10 minutes

RECIPE INGREDIENTS
◀ 5 egg whites, scrambled (free range if possible)
◀ ½ cup heated veggies, chopped (choose your favorite)
◀ Green onions, chopped, to taste
◀ ½ avocado, sliced
◀ ½ tomato (fresh, medium sized)
◀ 2 whole spelt or brown rice tortillas
◀ Salsa to taste

DIRECTIONS

Stir the first 5 ingredients together. Heat tortillas on a dry skillet for approximately 30 seconds on each side.

Scoop half the filling mixture into each tortilla and roll like a burrito.

Enjoy with fresh salsa on top.

Banana Walnut Oatmeal

RECIPE INGREDIENTS (all organic)
◀ 2 cups soy or almond milk
◀ Pinch of sea salt
◀ 1 cup steel-cut oats
◀ 1 teaspoon cinnamon

◀ 1 ripe banana, sliced
◀ 1/2 cup chopped walnuts (or your choice of nuts)
◀ 2 tablespoons maple syrup (grade B), optional

DIRECTIONS

In a small saucepan, combine milk and salt; heat over medium heat until steaming hot, but not boiling. Add oats and cook, stirring until creamy, 10 to 15 minutes; if too dry, add more soy milk. Remove the pan from the heat and stir in sliced banana and cinnamon. Use maple syrup and nuts as garnish.

For faster cooking, soak the oats overnight; cooking time will be cut in half.

Arugula Omelet

RECIPE INGREDIENTS (all organic)
◀ 4 egg whites with 2 eggs yolks, beaten
◀ 2 cups finely chopped arugula or spinach
◀ 1 cup grated Parmesan cheese (optional)
◀ Pinch cayenne pepper (optional)
◀ Pinch salt
◀ 2 tablespoons coconut oil
◀ 2 tablespoons grape seed oil

Directions

Mix the eggs, arugula, cheese, cayenne pepper, and salt until well mixed. In a sauté pan, heat coconut oil and grape seed oil over medium heat. Place about a quarter cup of the mixture in the pan for each omelet. Sauté until golden on both sides. Place on a warm plate. Serve with a slice of fresh tomato.

Vanilla Blueberry/Banana Bread

RECIPE INGREDIENTS (all organic)
- 1 1/3 cup plus 1 teaspoon whole spelt flour
- 1/2 teaspoon salt
- 1/2 teaspoon baking soda

1/4 teaspoon baking powder
- 2 tablespoons coconuts oil, room temperature
- 1/2 cup maple syrup
- 2 eggs
- 1 cup yogurt
- 1 teaspoon vanilla
- 1 banana, peeled and mashed
- 1/2 cup frozen blueberries

DIRECTIONS

Preheat the oven to 350°F and grease loaf pan. Combine all dry ingredients and mix well.

In a separate large bowl, combine butter and maple syrup and beat on high for 2 minutes. Gradually incorporate mixture of dry ingredients, followed by the yogurt and vanilla, eggs and mashed banana.

In a small bowl toss frozen blueberries with flour to coat and gently fold into the batter. Pour batter into greased loaf pan and bake for 50-60 minutes, or until a toothpick inserted into the center comes out clean. Let cool on a baking rack before removing pan.

Breakfast Parfait

RECIPE INGREDIENTS (all organic)
- cups chopped fresh pineapple
- firm, medium banana, peeled and sliced
- 1/3 cup chopped dates
- 1/3 cup chopped almonds, soaked overnight and peeled

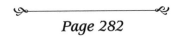

◄ 1 cup fresh raspberries (or other berries)
1 ◄ cup plain yogurt

DIRECTIONS
Build up your parfait in a wine glass as colorful as you like.

Baked French Toast

RECIPE INGREDIENTS (all organic)
◄ 1 loaf sourdough bread (cubed)
◄ 8 ounce package light cream cheese, diced
◄ 1 cup fresh blackberries (or any other berries)
◄ 12 egg whites and 5 eggs yolks
◄ 4 tablespoons olive oil
◄ 3 tablespoons maple syrup
◄ 2 teaspoons vanilla extract
◄ 2 cups soy milk
◄ 1/2 cup brown sugar
◄ 2 tablespoons cornstarch
◄ 1 cup water
◄ 1 tablespoon coconut oil

DIRECTIONS
Place half of the bread cubes in a lightly greased (with olive oil) 9-by-13-inch baking pan. Mix cream cheese with blueberries and remaining bread. In a large bowl, beat together eggs, soy milk, vanilla, and maple syrup. Pour egg mixture over bread. Cover pan and refrigerate overnight.

The next morning, remove pan from refrigerator 30 minutes before baking. Preheat oven to 350°F.

Cover cast iron pan with aluminum foil and bake in preheated oven for 30 minutes. Uncover pan and bake for an additional 30 minutes, until golden brown.

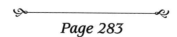

To make sauce: In a saucepan, combine sugar and cornstarch; add water. Boil over medium heat for 3 minutes, stirring constantly. Stir in blueberries and reduce heat. Simmer 8 to 10 minutes, or until the berries have burst. Stir in coconut oil. Serve the sauce over squares of French toast.

Scones

RECIPE INGREDIENTS (all organic)
- 1 cup brown rice flour
- 1 cup whole wheat or spelt flour
- 1/4 cup brown sugar
- 1/2 teaspoon salt
- 1 tablespoon baking powder (aluminum free)
- 1 tablespoon baking soda
- 1 1/4 cups plain yogurt
- 1 cup berries (your choice), frozen
- 3 tablespoons coconut oil

DIRECTIONS
Preheat the oven to 425°F. Combine the flours, baking powder, soda, salt, and sugar in a bowl, stirring with a fork to mix well. Add in the yogurt and frozen blueberries and continue to stir with a fork. The dough will become very sticky and will hold together in a rough mass. Lightly flour a cutting board and transfer the dough to it. Knead the dough 5 or 6 times and form into a circle about 10 inches around. For the glaze, spread the coconut oil over the top and the sides of the circle and sprinkle sugar on top. Cut the circle into 12 wedges and place each wedge on a non-stick cookie sheet, allowing about an inch between pieces. Bake for about 15 minutes, or until golden brown.

Avocado and Tangerine Salad

RECIPE INGREDIENTS
- 2 large avocados, sliced into thin wedges
- 4 tomatoes, cut into wedges
- 2 to 4 tangerines, peeled and cut into segments
- 1 red onion, sliced very thin
- 2 heads of baby lettuce or romaine hearts
- 2 tablespoons fresh chopped cilantro

Dressing

RECIPE INGREDIENTS
- 1/2 cup olive oil
- Juice of half a lemon
- Juice of one lime
- 2 garlic cloves, mashed or pressed
- 1 teaspoon dry mustard
- 1/4 teaspoon cayenne pepper
- 1/2 teaspoon honey
- Sea salt and pepper to taste

DIRECTIONS
Mix the dressing ingredients well in a blender until smooth.
On a plate lay the lettuce down. Arrange the avocado, tomato, tangerine, and onion slices on top. Pour over the dressing and garnish with fresh chopped cilantro.

Marinated Tomato

RECIPE INGREDIENTS
- 1 1/2 cups chopped tomatoes
- 1 clove garlic, mashed

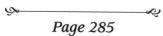

◀ 1 tablespoon fresh Italian parsley, chopped
◀ 1 tablespoon balsamic vinegar
◀ 1 tablespoon extra virgin olive oil
◀ Salt and pepper to taste
◀ 1 pound mixed greens

DIRECTIONS
Mix gently all ingredients (except mixed greens) and let marinate for 1/2 hour. Serve on bed of mixed greens.
This mix is also great on grilled fish.

Salad dressing

RECIPE INGREDIENTS
◀ 1/4 cup chardonnay, reduced over medium heat until half and cooled
◀ 1/4 cup extra virgin olive oil
◀ 1 shallot, chopped fine or mashed
◀ 1 whole lemon, juiced
◀ 1 teaspoon Dijon mustard
◀ 1 teaspoon chopped fresh tarragon
◀ Salt and pepper to taste
◀ 1 teaspoon raspberry jam
DIRECTIONS
Blend all the ingredients for the dressing together. Toss your choice of salad mixture and lightly pour on the dressing.

Spicy Chicken Chili

RECIPE INGREDIENTS
◀ 2 tablespoons grape seed oil
◀ 1 organic onion, chopped

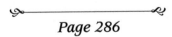

◀ 2 cloves organic garlic, minced
◀ 1 pound organic skinless chicken breast (about 4), cut into thin strips
◀ 4 teaspoons organic chili powder
◀ 1/4 tablespoon organic ground cumin
◀ 2 teaspoons fresh organic oregano
◀ 1 teaspoon sea salt (or to taste)
◀ 1-2 jalapeno peppers, seeds and ribs removed, chopped
◀ 1 1/2 cups canned organic crushed tomatoes with their juice (unsweetened)
◀ 2 1/2 cups organic chicken broth or homemade stock
   (make sure it is sugar free)
◀ 1 2/3 cups organic red beans (cook either dry beans or purchase frozen)
◀ 1 2/3 cups organic black beans (cook either dry beans or purchase frozen)
(Note: if you are cooking dry beans you must soak them for 24 hours without any salt in filtered water; this will release the gases that are in beans.)
◀ 1/2 teaspoon fresh-ground black pepper
◀ 1/3 cup chopped cilantro (optional)
◀ 1 teaspoon paprika

DIRECTIONS
   In a large saucepan, heat the oil over moderately low heat. Add the onion and garlic; cook until they start to soften, about 3 minutes. Increase the heat to medium and stir in the chicken strips. Cook until they are no longer pink, about 2 minutes. Stir in the chili powder, cumin, oregano, pepper, paprika, cilantro, and sea salt. Add the jalapeno, the tomatoes with their juice, and the chicken broth. Add your beans and bring to a boil, reduce the heat, cover, and simmer for 50-60 minutes, then serve.
   Serves 4

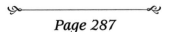

Chicken Wild Rice Soup

RECIPE INGREDIENTS
- 4-6 mixed pieces of bone-in skinless chicken (organic)
- 1 small organic onion, diced
- 2 teaspoons sea salt, or to taste
- ½ teaspoon cracked pepper
- 48 ounces filtered water
- 2 large organic carrots, sliced
- 3-4 stalks organic celery
- 1 cup organic wild rice blend
- Fresh organic sage and thyme leaves
- Organic chicken stock (no sugar added)

DIRECTIONS

Wash the chicken and place it in the crock pot along with the diced onion. Add the sea salt and pepper and cover with filtered water until the pot is about 1/2 to 2/3 full, depending on the size of your crock pot. For more flavors, include 2 cups organic chicken stock (no sugar added). Turn the pot on high until the water comes to a boil, and then reduce heat to low. Cook for about 3-4 hours or until the meat easily falls off the bone. Remove the chicken from the pot and add the vegetables, rice, and herbs. When the meat cools, take out the bones and tear the meat into smaller pieces and place it back in the pot. Turn the heat up to high and cook for another 2 hours or until the rice is soft. Serve hot and refrigerate or freeze the rest.

Pumpkin Soup

RECIPE INGREDIENTS
- 4-5 pound pumpkin, cleaned and cut into quarters
- 2 tablespoons olive oil
- Salt and pepper

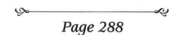

Directions

To cook pumpkin, place on a baking sheet. Spread with olive oil and salt and pepper. Bake in a 350°F oven for 1/2 hour or until fork-tender. Remove from oven. Cool. Scrape the flesh from the skin and reserve.

For the soup:
◀ 1 tablespoon grape seed oil
◀ 1 tablespoon fresh ginger, chopped
◀ 1 large onion, chopped
◀ 2 cloves garlic, chopped
◀ 4 cups chicken broth
◀ 1 teaspoon curry powder
◀ 1 teaspoon fresh nutmeg
◀ Sea salt to taste
◀ Sour cream or yogurt (optional)
◀ 2 tablespoons fresh cilantro, chopped

Directions

In a large sauce pan, sauté the onion, ginger, and garlic in the grape seed oil until soft. Add the curry powder and cook a few more minutes to release the flavor of the curry. Add the chicken broth and simmer for 3 to 4 minutes. Stir in the pumpkin and add salt to taste. Blend nutmeg with the soup until smooth. Pour into bowls and garnish with a small scoop of sour cream (optional) and fresh cilantro.

Asparagus Soup

RECIPE INGREDIENTS
◀ 2 bunches asparagus, chopped
◀ ½ cup cheese, grated (optional)
◀ 4 cups rice milk

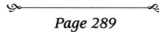

- ¼ cup brown rice
- ¼ cup basil
- 1 teaspoon celery salt
- 1 medium potato, chopped
- 1 teaspoon sea salt
- 3 tablespoons coconut oil (extra virgin)
- Pinch of ground pepper
- 1 yellow onion, chopped
- 1 clove garlic
- ½ cup mushrooms (oyster), sliced
- 1/8 cup Italian parsley
- ¼ cup chopped asparagus tips (set aside for use later)

Directions

1. Simmer rice and chopped potato in 2 cups rice milk. If needed, add more milk. After 15 minutes, add chopped asparagus, basil, celery salt, and pepper to taste. Simmer until vegetables are tender and let cool.

2. Saute onion, garlic, mushrooms, and reserved asparagus tips with a pinch of salt and parsley in 1 tablespoon coconut oil. Add to cooled broth and vegetables in blender or food processor and puree, slowly adding the 2 cups of rice milk. Can be served cold or hot.

LEEK SOUP

RECIPE INGREDIENTS
- 2 stocks of leek
- 2 medium potatoes
- 1 medium onion, chopped
- 4 cloves garlic, chopped
- 1 teaspoons turmeric powder
- 6 cups vegetable broth
- 2 tablespoons grape seed oil (for your cooking pan)

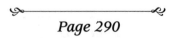

◀ Sea salt and pepper to taste

DIRECTIONS

In a large saucepan, heat the oil over moderately low heat. Add the onion, garlic, and turmeric. Cook until they start to soften, about 5-7 minutes. Add your potatoes to the pan and cook until soft. Sauté finely chopped leeks in the pan until softened. Add the vegetable broth to pan and salt and pepper to taste. Simmer for 15 minutes. Next pour the soup mixture into a blender or food processor and blend until all the lumps are gone and the soup is smooth. Serve once blended.

Quick Asian Soup

RECIPE INGREDIENTS
◀ 1 cup bean sprouts
◀ 1 cup carrots, chopped thin
◀ 1 cup chopped cabbage
◀ 1/2 cup chopped ginger
◀ 1 cup chopped lemon grass
◀ 1 cup chopped tofu
◀ 1 cup chopped celery
◀ 1 cup chopped parsley
◀ 1 cup chopped cilantro (don't chop fine, leave it leafy)
◀ 1 cup chopped mushroom (choose your favorite)
◀ 1 pinch of cayenne pepper (if desired for spicy soup)

DIRECTIONS

Get out your favorite soup bowl (or bowls if you are serving to other people). Simply add 1 tablespoon of each of the above listed ingredients into your bowl. Next pour boiling chicken broth into the bowl over the vegetables. Add a pinch of cayenne if desired to make your soup spicy. You can also use meso broth or vegetable broth in substitution for the chicken broth. You can also make your chicken broth from scratch. Store remaining chopped vegetables and soup broth in the fridge and use later to make quick Asian soup.

Chicken Fajita Salad

RECIPE INGREDIENTS
◀ 6 tablespoons grape seed oil
◀ 1/4 cup filtered water
◀ 2 tablespoons fresh organic parsley, minced
◀ 2 organic garlic cloves, minced
◀ 1 teaspoon organic ground cumin
◀ 1 teaspoon dried organic oregano
◀ 1-1/4 pounds boneless skinless chicken breasts, cut into 1-inch pieces
◀ 1 cup organic green onions, sliced
◀ 1 medium organic red bell pepper, julienned
◀ Shredded organic lettuce
◀ 2 medium organic tomatoes, cut into wedges
◀ 1 medium ripe organic avocado, peeled and sliced

DIRECTIONS
In a bowl, combine 4 tablespoons grape seed oil, water, parsley, garlic, cumin, and oregano. Pour half into a large bowl; add the chicken, turn to coat; refrigerate for 1 hour or overnight. Cover and refrigerate remaining marinade.

Drain and discard marinade from chicken. In a large skillet, sauté onions in remaining oil for 2 minutes. Add chicken; stir-fry for 2-3 minutes or until chicken just begins to brown. Add the red pepper and reserved marinade; stir-fry for 2 minutes.

Place lettuce on individual plates; top with chicken mixture, tomatoes, and avocado.

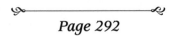

Add Green Chili Sauce to top of salad if desired (see recipe below)

Green Chili Sauce (gluten-free, nut-free, soy-free)

RECIPE INGREDIENTS
- 2 pounds fresh roasted or frozen roasted green chilies
- 10 – tomatillos
- 1 bunch cilantro, finely chopped
- ½ bunch Italian parsley
- 6 to 8 green onions
- 14 ounce can organic unsweetened chicken broth
- Sea salt to taste
- 1 teaspoon granulated garlic

DIRECTIONS
In a food processor, add the chilies, cilantro, onions, and tomatillos, then pulse to a medium puree (still some small chunks remaining). Transfer to a stock pot, add the broth and simmer for about 2 hours, cooking off some of the liquid. Add garlic and sea salt during the last 30 minutes to taste.

Guacamole

RECIPE INGREDIENTS
- 1 small fresh organic tomato
- 2-3 cloves garlic, minced
- Big pinch sea salt
- Small jalapeno
- 3 avocados
- 1/2 cup cilantro, chopped

DIRECTIONS
Mash/blend together.

PICO DE GALLO

RECIPE INGREDIENTS
- 8-10 Roma tomatoes
- 1/2-1 red onion (to taste)
- 1 jalapeno pepper (or more to taste)
- 2 medium cloves garlic
- Juice of one lime (if allowed on your detox plan)
- 1 tablespoon olive oil
- 4 tablespoons fresh cilantro, chopped
- 1 teaspoon coarse salt
- 1/2 teaspoon fresh ground black pepper

DIRECTIONS
   Start by dicing tomatoes and place into a medium sized bowl. Chop onion, jalapeno, and garlic to a fine consistency and place in the bowl with tomatoes. Add the fresh cilantro, salt, pepper, olive oil, and lime to the tomatoes. Mix well. Cover and refrigerate for at least 3 hours. Best if served the next day. Serve with organic corn tortilla chips, burritos, tacos, or any salad. As with any dish, you may add or delete ingredients to suit your personal taste or food restrictions specific to your detox plan.

Stuffed Bell Peppers

RECIPE INGREDIENTS
- 4 green, red, or yellow bell peppers
- 3 tablespoons grape seed oil
- 4 cloves of garlic, finely chopped
- 1 medium yellow onion, peeled and chopped
- 1 pound ground turkey (or for vegetarian, add one pound firm tofu, diced)
- 3 teaspoons salt
- 1 tablespoon granulated garlic

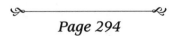

◀ 1 cup of cooked rice or cooked split peas (make sure that you precook your rice or split peas)
◀ 1 tablespoon turmeric
◀ 1 small can tomato paste
◀ 1/2 teaspoon fresh ground pepper
◀ 2 cups mushrooms (any type)

DIRECTIONS

1 Get a large sauté pan and add the grape seed oil to it, turning the stove top on medium heat. Add 1 medium yellow onion, chopped, into the pan and cook over medium heat until softened, then add your chopped garlic. Let the garlic and onion cook about 5-10 minutes; you want them to be soft and lightly golden brown. Next add one pound of ground turkey to the pan (or tofu) along with 3 teaspoons sea salt, ½ teaspoon fresh ground pepper, and 1 tablespoon turmeric; sauté all ingredients together for 10-15 min. Add in your mushrooms, adding 1 tablespoon granulated garlic to the pan, and cook with other ingredients until mushrooms are soft. Next add 1 small can of organic tomato paste to mixture, fill the empty tomato paste can four times with water, and pour into the mixture. Mix the tomato paste and added water with the mixture and let simmer for 20 minutes. Once it has cooked add in the already cooked rice (just mix the rice into the mixture, because the rice has already been cooked, you do not need to sauté it with the other ingredients); remove from the heat and set aside.

Preheat oven to 375°F. Meanwhile, cut tops off peppers, 1 inch from the stem end, and remove seeds. Arrange cut-side up in a Pyrex baking dish and then stuff peppers with filling you set aside from earlier. Use foil to cover the top of the baking dish, making sure the foil forms a good seal. You want the peppers to steam themselves and get soft. There is no need to add water or oil to the bottle of the baking dish; the pepper skin will be enough protection.

Place in oven and bake for 40-50 minutes (or longer, depending on how big the peppers are that you are stuffing).

Serves 4-6 (depending on size of peppers)

Garbanzo Bean Burger Wraps

RECIPE INGREDIENTS
◄ 15 ounces of organic frozen garbanzo beans, rinsed and drained
◄ 1 red bell pepper, finely chopped
◄ 1 carrot, grated
◄ 3 cloves garlic, minced
◄ 1 red chili pepper, seeded and minced
◄ 2 tablespoons chopped fresh cilantro
◄ Salt and black pepper to taste
◄ 1 teaspoon olive oil (optional)
◄ Butter lettuce or large leaf lettuce
◄ Tomatoes
◄ Onion

DIRECTIONS
Place garbanzo beans in the bowl of a food processor with bell pepper, carrot, garlic, red chili pepper, cilantro, sea salt, and pepper. Place the lid on the food processor, and pulse 5 times, then scrape the sides and pulse the mixture until it is evenly mixed. If the mixture looks dry, add olive oil.

Refrigerate garbanzo bean burger mixture for 30 minutes.

Preheat an oven to 350°F (175°C). Prepare a baking sheet with parchment paper or lightly grease with grape seed oil.

Shape the chilled garbanzo bean burger mixture into patties.

Bake 20 minutes, then carefully flip burgers and bake 10 more minutes, or until evenly browned.

Once cooked, take the garbanzo patty and wrap it with a large leaf of lettuce, add tomato, onion, and pickle to the wrap and you have garbanzo bean burger wraps.

Grilled Snapper

RECIPE INGREDIENTS
◀ 1 snapper per person
◀ 1/4 cup grape seed oil
◀ Juice of one lemon
◀ 2 garlic cloves, mashed
◀ 1/4 cup white wine
◀ 2 tablespoons chopped cilantro
◀ 1 tablespoon salt, and pepper to taste
DIRECTIONS
   Mix ingredients together; baste your fish for 20 minutes and grill over medium heat for about 10 minutes each side, basting often.

Fruit Salsa

RECIPE INGREDIENTS (all organic)
◀ cup papaya, finely diced
◀ cup pineapple, finely diced
◀ cup red bell peppers, finely diced
◀ cup green peppers, finely diced
◀ cup yellow peppers, finely diced
◀ cup red onions, finely diced
◀ 1 teaspoon jalapeno peppers, cleaned and finely chopped
◀ 1 tablespoon spring onions, sliced
◀ 6 pieces mint leaves, roughly chopped
◀ 1/2 cup olive oil
◀ 1 lime, juiced
◀ Salt and freshly ground pepper
◀ Garnish
◀ 4 cups sweet potato or taro chips

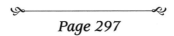

DIRECTIONS

Combine all ingredients in a bowl, mix coarsely, and season to taste with salt and pepper.

Place into serving bowls and serve with sweet potato or taro chips.

Beet Salad

RECIPE INGREDIENTS (all organic)
- 1 cup beets, cooked or baked (medium chopped)
- 2 small bunches arugula
- 4 teaspoons white-wine vinegar
- 1/2 cup olive oil (extra virgin)
- 1/4 cup nuts of your choice (roasted)
- Salt and pepper to taste

DIRECTIONS

Mix all the ingredients in a small bowl and chill for two hours. Put your arugula on the center of your plate and your mix over the top.

Fresh Grilled Vegetables (asparagus, zucchini)

RECIPE INGREDIENTS (all organic)
- 1 pound fresh asparagus or zucchini
- 2 tablespoons extra virgin coconut oil
- Salt to taste
- Freshly ground black pepper to taste

DIRECTIONS

Preheat barbecue. Clean and trim the asparagus or zucchini. Place in a shallow dish and sprinkle with oil, salt, and black pepper. Lay asparagus or other vegetables directly on the barbecue crosswise. Grill over medium heat about 3 minutes per side. Serve with lemon wedges.

Chicken Marcela

RECIPE INGREDIENTS (all organic)
- 2 pounds chicken breast
- 2 tablespoons olive oil
- 2 cloves garlic, mashed or pressed
- 1 teaspoon Italian parsley, chopped
- 1 teaspoon rosemary, chopped
- 1/4 cup Marcela wine
- 1 teaspoon salt and fresh ground pepper
- 1/2 teaspoon dry mustard

DIRECTIONS
   Mix all ingredients thoroughly and marinate chicken breast for one hour. Over medium heat, grill 4 minutes per side. Slice and serve with a green vegetable.

Pasta with Chard Sauce

RECIPE INGREDIENTS (all organic)
- 1/2 cup pine nuts
- 1 pound chard (spinach if chard not available), chopped
- 1 tangerine or orange
- 1 lime
- 1 pound fettuccine or linguine pasta (rice or soy)
- 1/4 cup grape seed oil
- 1/4 cup olive oil (virgin)
- 1 teaspoon garlic, chopped
- 2 large or 4 medium roasted beets, cut into 1/2-inch cubes
- 4 ounces feta or Gorgonzola cheese (optional)
- Salt and freshly ground pepper to taste

DIRECTIONS
   Toast the pine nuts in a 350°F oven for 10 minutes or until light brown. Cool. Wash the chard thoroughly, stem, and chop the leaves

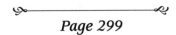

coarsely. Juice the tangerine and the lime into a measuring cup (about 1/2 cup of juice). Use fresh pasta if you can, which needs to boil for only a minute or two — dry pasta cooks longer (5 minutes); prepare the sauce before you cook the pasta. In a very large sauté pan, heat the grape seed oil and the garlic over a medium flame just until the garlic starts to color. Add the beets and citrus juice, and season with two large pinches of salt and some pepper. Boil until the liquid is reduced by about half. Add the greens and olive oil and toss. Drain the pasta and add it to the sauce, along with most of the pine nuts, and stir. Serve on warm plates with the extra pine nuts and half the cheese crumbled on top.

Cranberry Sauce

RECIPE INGREDIENTS
- ◀ 1 pound fresh cranberries, cooked
- ◀ 2 tablespoons blackberry or raspberry jam (sugar-free)
- ◀ 1/4 teaspoon fresh ginger, grated
- ◀ 1/3 cup red onion, diced
- ◀ 1/2 fresh orange juice
- ◀ Pinch of cayenne pepper

Directions
Mix other ingredients into the cranberries and refrigerate before serving.

Herb Baste

RECIPE INGREDIENTS
- ◀ 2 cloves garlic
- ◀ 1 cup Italian parsley, fresh
- ◀ 1 cup basil, fresh
- ◀ Salt and pepper to taste

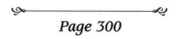

◀ 1 lemon, juiced
◀ 1/8 cup white wine (your choice)
◀ 1/8 cup extra virgin olive oil

Directions
    Place all in a blender and blend until smooth.
    This sauce is good for any type of meats before grilling.

Marinating Sauce (for red meat or lamb)

RECIPE INGREDIENTS (all organic)
◀ 4 tablespoons olive oil
◀ 1/8 cup red wine
◀ 3 cloves garlic, finely chopped
◀ 1 tablespoon fresh rosemary, chopped
◀ 1 tablespoon fresh thyme, chopped
◀ 1 tablespoon Italian parsley, chopped
◀ 1/2 tablespoon dry mustard
◀ Splash Worcestershire sauce
◀ Salt and pepper to taste
◀ Freshly grated horseradish

Directions
    Mix all of the ingredients and marinate your meat for 20 minutes before grilling.

Sautéed Green Beans with Nuts and Mango

RECIPE INGREDIENTS (all organic)
◀ 1 pound fresh green beans
◀ 1 cup mango
◀ 2 tablespoons coconut oil

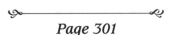

◀ 2 cloves garlic, thinly sliced
1/4 cup Champaign vinegar
1/8 cup sliced roasted almonds or pine nuts

Directions
    Blanch the green beans in salted boiling water and drain in cold water. In a large saucepan over medium high heat, add coconut oil, green beans, and garlic and sauté for 2 minutes. Mix mango and vinegar. Serve with sliced toasted spelt bread and your choice of nuts sprinkled on top.

Orzo with Asparagus

RECIPE INGREDIENTS (all organic)
◀ 1 medium onion, sliced
◀ 1 small fennel, sliced
◀ 2 cloves garlic, chopped
◀ 1/8 cup grape seed oil
◀ 2 teaspoons extra virgin coconut oil
◀ Pinch of sea salt
◀ 2 teaspoons fresh Parmesan cheese (optional)
◀ Pinch of red pepper flakes
◀ 1/4 teaspoon fresh thyme
◀ 1 pound orzo
◀ 1 quart chicken stock
◀ 1/2 to 1 pound asparagus, cut at angle

Directions
    In a high sauce pan, heat grape seed and coconut oils over medium heat. Add onion, fennel, and garlic and sauté until very soft. Add orzo and sauté for a minute; add 1/2 cup chicken stock. Stir as you would risotto until liquid is absorbed. Repeat until pasta is almost al dente. Add asparagus and simmer until tender. Top with Parmesan, pepper flakes, and thyme.

Apricot Chicken Curry

RECIPE INGREDIENTS (all organic)
- 1 cup onion, chopped
- 1 teaspoon garlic, minced
- 1 teaspoon sea salt
- 3 teaspoons coconut oil
- 2 teaspoons grape seed oil
- 1 tablespoon grated fresh ginger
- 1/2 cup orange juice
- 1/2 teaspoon grape seed oil
- 1/2 teaspoon curry powder
- 1/8 teaspoon sesame oil
- 1/2 teaspoon rice vinegar
- 1 tablespoon light soy sauce
- 1/2 cup soaked apricots, chopped
- 2 tablespoons fresh cilantro, chopped
- 2 pounds whole chicken meat, sliced (dark and white)
- 2 cups wild and brown rice, mixed
- 1/4 cup extra virgin olive oil

Directions

In large pan, melt the coconut oil with grape seed oil add onion until half cooked; add garlic and curry, then add the chicken and cook until golden brown.

In a saucepan combine ginger, orange juice, grape seed oil, sesame oil, rice vinegar, wine, soy sauce, apricot, and cilantro. Bring to a simmer. Add to the chicken and cook in the oven at 350°F for 20 minutes. Serve over the rice. (Start cooking the rice as the same time.)

Cook the rice with water for 30 minutes with 1 teaspoon sea salt and 1/4 cup olive oil until done.

Chicken Orange Thyme

RECIPE INGREDIENTS (all organic)
- 1 chicken, cut into 8 pieces
- 4 spring onions, sliced thick
- 1 cup white wine (dry)
- 4 tablespoons olive oil
- 1 tablespoon fresh thyme
- 1/2 teaspoon lemon rind, grated
- 1/2 cup orange juice
- Salt and pepper

Directions

Rub chicken pieces with salt and pepper. Heat olive oil in a pan, add chicken pieces, and sauté them on one side till golden brown. Turn over, add spring onions and rosemary, and sauté for another 4 minutes. Pour in the white wine and let it reduce for 3 minutes; add broth, reduce flame, cover, and gently cook for about 40 minutes. At the end of simmering time, add the lemon rind.

Side dish: brown rice or saffron rice

Smoked Salmon Tartar

RECIPE INGREDIENTS
- 1 pound smoked salmon, diced small
- 1/2 cup cucumber, finely diced
- 2 shallots, finely diced
- 1 teaspoon cilantro
- 1/3 cup chive, finely diced

Season with salt (if needed), black pepper, and Lea & Perrins sauce. Mix the diced salmon well with the cucumber, shallots, and chives and season as necessary. Mold into a round disk.

Pan Seared Salmon

RECIPE INGREDIENTS
- 12 ounces salmon, cut into four 3-ounce squares
- Sea salt to taste
- Coarse ground coriander to taste
- Extra virgin olive oil to taste
- 1 clove garlic, pressed

Directions
Season salmon with salt, garlic, coriander, and extra virgin olive oil; preheat the pan and sear in a moderately heated pan until meat is crispy; turn and place in a 375°F oven for approximately 3 minutes to complete the cooking. Serves 2 small or appetizer-size servings.

Fava Bean Dip

RECIPE INGREDIENTS
- 2 cups fava beans (outer skin removed), cooked
- 3 cloves garlic, mashed
- 1 cup of onion (yellow)
- 1/8 teaspoon hot paprika
- 1/8 teaspoon ground cumin
- 1 whole lime, juiced
- Salt and pepper to taste
- 1/4 cup extra virgin olive oil

Directions
Sauté onion with garlic until golden brown. Put all ingredients into a bowl or a food processor. Either hand mash or blend until smooth (you may need to add more olive oil to make it smooth). Serve in a bowl with vegetables; sprinkle with fresh chopped Italian parsley.

Eggplant Tofu Casserole

RECIPE INGREDIENTS
- ½ cup onion
- 1 teaspoon garlic, minced
- 2 cups eggplant
- 1 cup tofu
- 1 cup tomato, sliced
- 1 cup green pepper
- ¼ cup grape seed oil
- 1 teaspoon coconut oil
- ¼ cup soy ginger sauce
- ¼ cup warm water
- ¼ teaspoon pepper flakes
- Salt and pepper to taste

Directions

Using a cast iron skillet, add oil and sauté the onion over medium heat until golden. Add garlic, then add eggplant and stir until half cooked. Add tofu and the rest of the ingredients and cook for 10 minutes. Add soy ginger and water at the end and cook for 5 more minutes. Serve with brown rice or side dish.

Easy Vegan Spelt Pie Crust

RECIPE INGREDIENTS
- 3 cups spelt flour (not sprouted)
- 1 teaspoon sea salt
- 1/2 cup organic soy milk (unsweetened)
- 1/2 cup grape seed oil

DIRECTIONS

In a food processor add the spelt flour and salt, and process for a minute to incorporate.

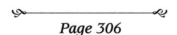

Combine the non-dairy milk and light oil in a cup and mix well. I use a whisk to do this. Then feed the milk-oil mixture through the feeding tube in the food processor and into the flour mixture. The dough should be in large crumbles. At this point, stop the machine and feel the dough. It shouldn't be sticky or dry, but a little oily and holding together well. Try not to handle the dough too much as it tends to toughen the dough.

Once you have the right consistency, remove the dough crumbles onto a prepared surface to roll out your dough. I use a large plastic sheet, but waxed paper can also be used. I try to avoid using a floured surface as it will make the dough dry. I have found that with this dough that it isn't necessary.

Shape the dough into a disc and cut it in half. Reshape the first piece of dough into a disc and roll it out. I wrap the dough around my rolling pin then place it onto the pie pan and unroll. Once I have the dough in place, I position it carefully but do not stretch it; it will shrink. Prick the sides and bottom of the bottom crust.

Fill the pie with the desired ingredients and roll out the second disc of dough and put it on top.

Flute the edges with a fork and then trim the pie crust edges. Brush the pie with some of the non-dairy milk and then make slits in the top crust to let out the steam.

Bake according to the type of pie you are making.

Blueberry Filling for Pies

RECIPE INGREDIENTS
- 4 cups blueberries (fresh or frozen)
- 2 tablespoons organic agave nectar (if allowed on your detox plan)
- 1/4 cup lemon juice (if allowed on your detox plan)
- 1/4-1/3 cup non-aluminum cornstarch
  (depending on how thick you like your filling)
- 1/4 cup water

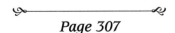

If you are on stage one of your detox plan and cannot have agave or lemon juice, simply make this recipe without those items; it will still taste great.

DIRECTIONS

In a heavy saucepan mix together blueberries, agave, and lemon juice.

Over medium heat bring to boil, stirring frequently. Mix cornstarch with water to make a paste. Pour into berry mixture, stirring constantly until thick.

Remove from heat and let cool. You can now freeze it or use for pie. Bake at 400°F for about 35 minutes.

References

- Karadinall, A. F. Association between beta-carotene and acute myocardial infarction depends upon polyunsaturated fatty acid status. The EURAMIC study. Arteriosclerosis, Thrombosis & Vascular Biology. 15(6):726-732, 1995.

- Simopoulos, A. P. The role of fatty acids in gene expression: health implications. Ann Nutr Metab. 40:303-311, 1996.

- Kris-Etherton, P. Summary of the Scientific Conference on Dietary Fatty Acids and Cardiovascular Health: Conference summary from the Nutrition Committee of the American Heart Association. Circulation. 103:1034-1039, 2001.

- Delport, R., et al. Antioxidant vitamins and coronary artery disease risk in South African males. Clin Chim Acta. 278:55-60, 1998.

- Haas, Elson M. Staying Healthy with Nutrition. Celestial Arts, Berkeley, California, USA. 1992:95.

- Bjelke. Dietary vitamin A and human lung cancer. Int J Cancer. 15(4):561-565, 1975.

Five-year follow-up results for 8,278 men who in mail surveys had reported their cigarette smoking and dietary habits showed: (1) an index for vitamin A intake to be negatively associated with lung cancer incidence at all levels of cigarette smoking;(2) this association to be more clearly expressed in the subset of histologically proven pulmonary carcinomas other than adenocarcinoma; and (3) the positive association between cigarette smoking and lung cancer to occur irrespective of the dietary level of vitamin A or related factors.

- Hsing, A. W., et al. Serologic precursors of cancer. Retinol, carotenoids, and tocopherol and the risk of prostate cancer. Journal of the National Cancer Institute. 82(11):941-946, 1990.

The authors investigated the associations of serum retinol, the carotenoids beta-carotene and lycopene, and tocopherol (vitamin E) with the risk of prostate cancer in a nested case-control study. For the study, serum obtained in 1974 from 25,802 persons in Washington County, MD, was used. Serum levels of the nutrients in 103 men who developed prostate cancer during the subsequent 13 years were compared with levels in 103 control subjects matched for age and race. Although no significant associations were observed with beta-carotene, lycopene, or tocopherol, the data suggested an inverse relationship between serum retinol and risk of prostate cancer. The authors analyzed data on the distribution of serum retinol by quartiles, using the lowest quartile as the reference value. Odds ratios were 0.67, 0.39, and 0.40 for the second, third, and highest quartiles, respectively.

- Cohen, B.E., et al. Reversal of postoperative immunosuppression in man by vitamin A. Surg Gynecol Obstet. 149:658-62, 1979.

The effects of therapy with vitamin A on immune responsiveness after extensive surgical treatment were studied in vitro. Postoperatively, in control patients, there was depression of the total lymphocyte count and the response in the mixed lymphocyte reaction to a pool of stimulating cells. Treatment with pharmacologic dosages of vitamin A prevented depression of these parameters in the postoperative period. The mitogenic response to phytohemagglutinin and monocyte mediated hemolysis was not consistently altered by operation in control patients, but there was a trend toward increased activity in those receiving vitamin A. Vitamin A appears to be an immunostimulant in man.

• Holford, P. Improve Your Digestion. Judy Piatkus (Publishers). London, United Kingdom. 1999:109.

• Berson, E. L., et al. A randomized trial of vitamin A and vitamin E supplementation for retinitis pigmentosa. Arch Ophthalmol. 111(6):761-772, 1993.

• Cutaneous vitamins A and E in the context of ultraviolet- or chemically-induced oxidative stress. Skin Pharmacology and Applied Skin Physiology. 14(6):363-372, 2002.

• Varosy, P. Meeting of the American Heart Association. Hawaii, USA, 2002.

Women over the age of 65 who used vitamin D had almost 33% less risk of dying from heart disease as women who did not take the supplements, the researchers told a meeting in Hawaii of the American Heart Association. Researchers followed 9,704 women aged 65 and older who were taking part in an osteoporosis study. Half the women were taking vitamin D supplements. After an average of 11 years, 420 of the women died of coronary heart disease. Women who took extra vitamin D supplements were 31 percent less likely to have died of heart disease than those who did not take the supplements. Vitamin D may be associated with reduced heart disease risk, as so-called hardening of the arteries (atherosclerosis) can progress from a buildup of fat in the blood vessels to calcification of that buildup. There is evidence suggesting that calcification in the arteries is very similar to the calcification process that occurs in bone. Women with osteoporosis tend to have more calcium in the walls of their arteries than women with normal bones. It is possible that the same hormonal processes that lead to calcium loss from bones may lead to accumulation of calcium in atherosclerotic plaques. The nature of the mechanism is unclear.

• Harries, A. D., et al. Vitamin D status in Crohn's disease: association with nutrition and disease activity. Gut. 26(11):1197-1203, 1985.

• Deluca, H. F., et al. Vitamin D: its role and uses in immunology. FASEB J. 15(14):2579-2585, 2001.

• Segala, M. (editor). Disease Prevention and Treatment 3rd Edition. Life Extension Media. Florida, USA. 2000:140.

High-dose (2,000 - 3,000 IU per day) vitamin D (vitamin D3) is recommended for cancer patients on the basis of its ability to induce cancer cell differentiation. This high dosage should be closely monitored by the patient's physician (monthly blood tests are required to confirm that vitamin D toxicity is not occurring).

- Lewis, R. D., et al. Nutrition, physical activity and bone health in women. International Journal of Sport Nutrition. 8(3):250-284, 1998.

- Isala, G., et al. High prevalence of hypovitaminosis D in female type 2 diabetic population. Diabetes Care. 24(8):1496, 2001.

- Gloth, F. M. 3rd, et al. Vitamin D vs broad spectrum phototherapy in the treatment of seasonal affective disorder. J Nutr Health Aging 3(1):5-7, 1999.

- Acuff, R. V. Get the facts on natural vitamin E. Nature's Impact. February/March 1999:26-29.

- Christensen, F., et al. Acta Physiol Scand. 27:315, 1952.

- Hoffman La Roche corporation. Diabetes and vitamin E. Diabetes. 44(2), 1995.

- Bandt, M. D., et al. Vitamin E uncouples joint destruction and clinical inflammation in a transgenic mouse model of rheumatoid arthritis. Arthritis Rheum. 46(2):522-532, 2002.

- Thiele, J. J., et al. The antioxidant network of the stratum corneum. Curr Probl Dermatol. 29:26-42, 2001.

- Suttie, J. W. Vitamin K and human nutrition. Journal of the American Dietetic Association. (5):585-590, 1992.

- Chlebowski, R. T., et al. Vitamin K in the treatment of cancer. Cancer Treatment Review. 12:49-63, 1985.

- Hodges, S. J., et al. Circulating levels of vitamins K1 and K2 decreased in elderly women with hip fracture. J Bone Miner Res. 8(10):1241-1245, 1993.

- Leslie, D., et al. Is there a role for thiamine supplementation in the management of heart failure. American Heart Journal. 131(6):1248-1250, 1996.

- Du, S., et al. [Relationship between dietary nutrients intakes and human prostate cancer]. Wei Sheng Yen Chiu. 26(2):122-125, 1997.

- Agbayewa, M. O., et al. Pyridoxine, ascorbic acid and thiamine in Alzheimer and comparison subjects. Canadian Journal of Psychiatry 37(9):661-662, 1992.

- Roberts, A. J., et al. Nutraceuticals: the Complete Encyclopedia of Supplements, Herbs, Vitamins and Healing Foods. Berkely Publishing Group. New York, USA. 2001:225.

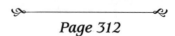

• Beales, P. E., et al. Diet can influence the ability of nicotinamide to prevent diabetes in the non-obese diabetic mouse: a preliminary study. Diabetes Metab Res Rev. 15(1):21-28, 1999.

• Folsom, A. R., et al. Prospective study of coronary heart disease incidence in relation to fasting total homocysteine, related genetic polymorphisms, and B vitamins: the Atherosclerosis Risk in Communities (ARIC) study. Circulation. 98(3):204-210, 1998.

• Folkers, K., et al. The activities of coenzyme Q10 and vitamin B6 for immune response. Biochem-Biophys Res Commun. 193(1):88-92, 1993.

• Brattstrom, L., et al. Pyridoxine reduces cholesterol and low-density lipoprotein and increases antithrombin III activity in 80-year-old men with low plasma pyridoxal 5-phosphate. Scand J Clin Lab Invest. 50(8):873-877, 1990.

• Haas, Elson M. Staying Healthy with Nutrition. Celestial Arts, Berkeley, California, USA. 1992:124.

• Dolby Toews, V. Brain Power. Health Journal News & Views. 3(5), 2000.

• Can reduced folic acid and vitamin B12 levels cause deficient DNA methylation producing mutations which initiate atherosclerosis? Med Hypotheses. 53(5):421-424, 1999.

• Campbell, R. E., et al. Vitamin B12 in the treatment of viral hepatitis. Am J Med Sci. 224:252-262, 1952.

• Barcikowska, M., et al. [Level of vitamin B12 and folic acid in blood serum of patients with senile dementia]. Wiad Lek. 47(9-10):346-351, 1994.

• Berglund, High-altitude training. Sports Med. 14:289-303, 1992.

• Komar, V. I. [The use of pantothenic acid preparations in treating patients with viral hepatitis A]. Ter Arkh. 63:58-60, 1991.

Calcium pantothenate (300 mg and 600 mg daily) and pantetheine (90 mg and 180 mg daily) were administered orally for 3-4 weeks as combined therapy in 156 patients with hepatitis A. A favorable clinical effect, as well as an enhanced immunomodulatory action, a beneficial effect on the level of blood serum immunoglobulins, and an increased phagocytic activity of peripheral blood neutrophils were reported. Pantetheine provided the most pronounced therapeutic effect.

• Mervyn, L. Thorsons Complete Guide to Vitamins and Minerals (2nd Edition). Thorsons Publishing Group, Wellingborough, England. 1989:58.

• Colombo, V. E., et al. Treatment of brittle fingernails and onychoschizia with biotin: scanning electron microscopy. J Am Acad Dermatol. 23(6 Part 1):1127-1132, 1990.

• Kelly, G. S. Insulin resistance: lifestyle and nutritional interventions. Alternative Medicine Review. 5(2):109-132, 2000.

• Malik, N. S., et al. Vitamins and analgesics in the prevention of collagen ageing. Age and Ageing. 25(4):279-284, 1996.

• Bordia, A. K. The effect of vitamin C on blood lipids, fibrinolytic activity and platelet adhesiveness in patients with coronary artery disease. Atherosclerosis. 35(2):181-187, 1980.

• Abel, B. Randomized trial of clomiphene citrate and vitamin C for male infertility. British Journal of Urology. 54(6):780-784, 1982.

• Cappuccio, F. P., et al. Does oral calcium supplementation lower high blood pressure? A double blind study. Journal of Hypertension 5(1):67-71, 1987.

• Burtis, W. J., et al. Dietary hypercalciuria in patients with calcium oxalate kidney stones. American Journal of Clinical Nutrition. 60:424-429, 1994.

Dietary salt, as assessed by urinary sodium excretion, rather than dietary calcium, was found to be the principal dietary factor influencing urinary calcium excretion. This indicates that the positive association between hypercalciuria and kidney stones is attributable to excessive dietary consumption of salt, rather than excessive consumption of calcium.

• Heaney, R. P., et al. Calcium and weight: clinical studies. Journal of the American College of Nutrition. 21(2), 2002.

• Nazar, K., et al. Phosphate supplementation prevents a decrease of triiodothyronine and increases resting metabolic rate during low energy diet. J Physiol Pharmacol. 47(2):373-383, 1996.

• Ralo, J. Magnesium: Another metal to bone up on. Science News. 154:134, 1998.

• Davis, W. H., et al. Monotherapy with magnesium increases abnormally low high density lipoprotein cholesterol: A clinical essay. Clin Ther Res. 36:341-346, 1984.

• Vayda, W. Are you a sugarholic? Australian Wellbeing. 17:85-93, 1986.

• Roberts, H. J., et al. Does aspartame cause human brain cancer? Journal of Advancement of Medicine. 4(4):231-241, 1991.

• Lipton, R. B., et al. Aspartame as a dietary trigger of headache. Headache. 29(2):90-92, 1989.

• Fowkes, S. Wm. Aspartame and multiple sclerosis?. Smart Drug News. 7(3):10-11, 1999.

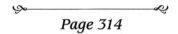

• Asthma from aspartame. Cortlandt Forum. 116:36-49, 1991.

• Gregus, Z, et al. Disposition of metals in rats: a comparative study of fecal, urinary, and biliary excretion and tissue distribution of eighteen metals. Toxicol Appl Pharmacol. 85:24-38, 1986.

• Sinclair, S., et al. Migraine headaches: nutritional, botanical and other alternative approaches. Alternative Medicine Review. 4(2):86-95, 1999.

• Murray, Michael T. The Encyclopedia of Nutritional Supplements: the essential guide for improving your health naturally. Prima Publishing, Rocklin, California, USA. 1996:24.

• Pearson, D. & Shaw, S. Life Extension: A Practical Scientific Approach. Warner Book, New York, NY, USA. 1982:195.